Prehospital Management of Acute STEMI

Practical Approaches and International Strategies for Early Intervention

The Cardiovascular Team Approach

A book series focusing on the interprofessional team approach for the management and prevention of cardiovascular diseases.

Editors-in-Chief:
Joseph S. Alpert, MD, FAHA, FACC, MACP, FESC
Lynne T. Braun, PhD, CNP, FAHA, FAAN
Barbara J. Fletcher, RN, MN, FAHA, FAAN
Gerald Fletcher, MD, FAHA, FACC, FACP

Look for these and other forthcoming series titles from Cardiotext Publishing.

Volume 1: *Heart Failure: Strategies to Improve Outcomes*
Ileana L. Piña, MD, MPH, FACC, FAHA, and
Elizabeth A. Madigan, PhD, RN, FAAN, editors

Volume 2: *Prehospital Management of Acute STEMI: Practical Approaches and International Strategies for Early Intervention*
Edgardo Escobar, MD, FACC, FAHA, and
Alejandro Barbagelata, MD, FAHA, FSCAI, editors

Volume 3: *Acute Coronary Syndrome: Urgent and Follow-up Care*
Eileen Handberg, PhD, ARNP, BC, FAHA, FACC, and
R. David Anderson, MD, MS, FACC, FSCAI, editors

Volume 4: *Atrial Fibrillation: A Multidisciplinary Approach to Improving Patient Outcomes*
N.A. Mark Estes III MD, FACC, FHRS, FAHA, FESC, and
Albert L. Waldo, MD, PhD (Hon), FACC, FHRS, FAHA, FACCP, editors

Please visit www.cardiotextpublishing.com for more information about this series.

Prehospital Management of Acute STEMI

Practical Approaches and International Strategies for Early Intervention

The Cardiovascular Team Approach Series

VOLUME 2

Edgardo Escobar, MD, FACC, FAHA
Alejandro Barbagelata, MD, FAHA, FSCAI
Volume Editors

Joseph S. Alpert, MD, FAHA, FACC, MACP, FESC
Lynne T. Braun, PHD, CNP, FAHA, FAAN
Barbara J. Fletcher, RN, MN, FAHA, FAAN
Gerald Fletcher, MD, FAHA, FACC, FACP
Editors-in-Chief

cardiotext.
PUBLISHING
Minneapolis, Minnesota

Cardiotext Publishing, LLC
3405 W. 44th Street
Minneapolis, Minnesota 55410
USA

www.cardiotextpublishing.com

Any updates to this book may be found at:
cardiotextpublishing.com/prehospital-management-of-acute-stemi

Comments, inquiries, and requests for bulk sales can be directed to the publisher at: info@cardiotextpublishing.com.

Library of Congress Control Number: 2015933408

ISBN: 978-1-935395-66-9

Printed in the United States of America

To my wife Josefina for her patience and to ITMS, Telemedicina for giving me the inspiration

—Edgardo Escobar

To my beloved wife and 3 beautiful children

—Alejandro Barbagelata

Contents

About the Editors-in-Chief

Editors-in-Chief

Joseph S. Alpert, MD, FAHA, FACC, MACP, FESC
Professor of Medicine, University of Arizona Health Science Network; Editor-in-Chief, *The American Journal of Medicine*, Tucson, Arizona

Lynne T. Braun, PhD, CNP, FAHA, FAAN
Professor, Department of Adult Health and Gerontological Nursing, Rush University College of Nursing; Nurse Practitioner, Section of Cardiology, Rush University Medical Center, Chicago, Illinois

Barbara J. Fletcher, RN, MN, FAHA, FAAN
Clinical Associate Professor, Brooks College of Health, School of Nursing, University of North Florida, Jacksonville, Florida

Gerald Fletcher, MD, FAHA, FACC, FACP
Professor in Medicine (Cardiovascular Diseases), Mayo Clinic College of Medicine, Mayo Clinic Florida, Jacksonville, Florida

About the Authors

Editors

Edgardo Escobar, MD, FACC, FAHA
Professor of Medicine, University of Chile; Medical Director, ITMS Telemedicine of Chile, Santiago, Chile

Alejandro Barbagelata, MD, FAHA, FSCAI
Associate Professor of Medicine, Division of Cardiology, University of Texas Medical Branch, Galveston, Texas

Contributors

George L. Adams, MD, MHS, FACC
Director of Cardiovascular and Peripheral Vascular Research, Rex Healthcare, Raleigh, North Carolina; Clinical Associate Professor of Medicine, University of North Carolina Health Systems, Chapel Hill, North Carolina

Zubair Ahmed, MD, FSCAI
Assistant Professor, Interventional Cardiology; Director, Cardiac Catheterization Laboratories, University of Arkansas for Medical Sciences, Little Rock, Arkansas

Salman J. Bandeali, MBBS
Cardiology Fellow, Texas Heart Institute, Houston, Texas

Yochai Birnbaum, MD
Professor of Medicine, Department of Medicine, Section of Cardiology, Baylor College of Medicine, Houston, Texas

Roberto Vieira Botelho, MD, PhD
Director, Triangulo Heart Institute, Uberlandia, Brazil

Qiangjun Cai, MD, FACC, FACP
Division of Cardiology, University of Texas Medical Branch, Galveston, Texas

Peter Clemmensen, MD, DMSc, FESC, FSCAI
Chair, Professor of Cardiology, University of Copenhagen; Chief Physician, Heart Centre, Rigshospitalet, Denmark, Copenhagen

Nicolas Danchin, MD, PhD, FESC
Department of Cardiology, Hôpital Européen Georges Pompidou, Assistance Publique Hôpitaux de Paris, and Université Paris Descartes, Paris, France

Eric Durand, MD, PhD
Department of Cardiology, University Hospital of Rouen, Rouen, France

Freij Gobal, MD
Cardiology, NEA Baptist Clinic, Jonesboro, Arkansas

Patrick Goldstein, MD
Medical Director, Head of Department, Emergency Department and SAMU, Lille University Hospital, Lille, France

Denise Greci Robinson, RN, MS, CNS
Clinical Nurse Specialist, Emergency Department, Stanford University Medical Center, Stanford, California

Liliana Grinfeld, MD, PhD, FSCAI, FACC
Interventional Cardiologist, Docent and Investigator, Cardiovascular Fisiopathology Institute, School of Medicine, University of Buenos Aires, Buenos Aires, Argentina

Abdul Hakeem, MBBS
Assistant Professor, Division of Cardiovascular Medicine, University of Arkansas, Little Rock, Arkansas

Timothy D. Henry, MD
Director, Division of Cardiology, Lee and Harold Kapelovitz Chair in Research Cardiology, Cedars-Sinai Heart Institute; Professor, Department of Medicine, Cedars-Sinai Medical Center; Professor In Residence, Step 3, David Geffen School of Medicine; Department of Medicine, University of California Los Angeles, Los Angeles, California

David A. Hildebrandt, RN, NREMTP
Minneapolis Heart Institute Foundation at Abbott Northwestern Hospital, Minneapolis, Minnesota

Henry D. Huang, MD
Clinical and Research Electrophysiology Fellow, Arrhythmia Service, Division of Cardiology, Beth Israel Deaconess Medical Center; Harvard Thorndike Electrophysiology Institute, Boston, Massachusetts

Waleed T. Kayani, MD
Department of Medicine, Baylor College of Medicine, Houston, Texas

Darren Knapp, EMT-P
Vital Heart Response, Cardiac Sciences, EDM Zone, Alberta Health Services; Mazankowski Alberta Heart Institute, Edmonton, Alberta, Canada

David M. Larson, MD, FACEP
Chairman, Department of Emergency Services, Ridgeview Medical Center, Waconia, Minnesota; Associate Clinical Professor, University of Minnesota Medical School Minneapolis, Minnesota

Michael J. Pompliano, NREMT, BS Biological Sciences
University of South Carolina Honors College, Columbia, South Carolina

Etienne Puymirat, MD
Department of Cardiology, Hôpital Européen Georges Pompidou, Université Paris Descartes, Paris, France

Florencia Rolandi, MD, MSc
Cardiology Department, Italian Hospital of Buenos Aires, Buenos Aires, Argentina

Maria Sejersten, MD, DMSc
Department of Cardiology, Roskilde Hospital, Roskilde, Denmark

Barry F. Uretsky, MD
Director, Interventional Cardiology, University of Arkansas for Medical Sciences and the Central Arkansas Veterans Health System, Little Rock, Arkansas

Thais Waisman, MD, PhD
Engineering School at University of São Paulo – Interlab-EPUSP, São Paulo, Brazil

Robert C. Welsh, MD, FRCPC, FACC, FAHA, FESC
Professor of Medicine, Department of Medicine and Division of Cardiology, Mazankowski Alberta Heart Institute and University of Alberta, Edmonton, Alberta, Canada

Eric Wiel, MD, PhD
Professor, Anesthesiologist-Intensivist-Emergency Physician, Deputy Head of the Emergency Department & Academic Head of Emergency Medicine, Emergency Department, Lille University Hospital; Public Health Laboratory (EA 2694), Northern France University, Lille, France

Abbreviations

ACC	American College of Cardiology
ACCF	American College of Cardiology Foundation
ACEIs	angiotensin converting enzyme inhibitors
ACLS	advanced cardiac life support
ACP	advanced care paramedic
ACS	acute coronary syndrome
ACTION	Acute Coronary Treatment and Intervention Outcomes Network
ADMIRAL	Abciximab before Direct Angioplasty and Stenting in Myocardial Infarction Regarding Acute and Long-Term Follow-Up
AEDs	automated external defibrillators
AHA	American Heart Association
AHS	Alberta Health Services
ALS	advanced life support
AMI	acute myocardial infarction
AMU	advanced emergency medical unit
ARVD	arrhythmogenic right ventricular dysplasia
ASSENT-3	Assessment of the Safety and Efficacy of a New Thrombolytic agent
BLS	basic life support
BRAVE	Bavarian Reperfusion AlternatiVes Evaluation
CA	cardiac arrest
CABG	coronary artery bypass grafting
CACI	Argentine College of Interventional Cardioangiologists
CAD	coronary artery disease
CAG	coronary angiography

CCL	cardiac catheterization laboratory
CCP	critical care paramedic
CCT RN	critical care transport nurse
CHD	coronary heart disease
CHF	congestive heart failure
CL	catheterization laboratory
CLA	catheterization laboratory activation
CMS	Centers for Medicare and Medicaid Services
CNS	clinical nurse specialists
CPR	cardiopulmonary resuscitation
cTnI	cardiac troponin I
CVDs	cardiovascular diseases
D2B	door-to-balloon
DANAMI-2	Danish trial in acute myocardial infarction-2
DDKM	Danish Healthcare Quality Program
DIDO	door-in to door-out
DTD	door-to-device
DTN	door-to-needle
ECG	electrocardiogram/electrocardiographic
ED	Emergency Department
EMR	emergency medical responder
EMS	emergency medical service/systems
EMT	emergency medical technician
ERC	European Resuscitation Council
ESC	European Society of Cardiology
FINESSE	Facilitated Intervention with Enhanced Reperfusion Speed to Stop Events
FMC	first medical contact
FTT	Fibrinolytic Therapy Trialists'
GDP	gross domestic product
GP	glycoprotein
GUSTO	Global Use of Strategies to Open Occluded Arteries in Acute Coronary Syndromes
GWTG	Get With the Guidelines
ILCOR	International Liaison Committee on Resuscitation
INDEC	National Institute of Statistics and Census [Argentina]

ISIS-2	International Study of Infarct Survival
ITMS	International Telemedical System SA
IVCD	intraventricular conduction delay
LBBB	left bundle branch block
LMWH	low molecular weight heparin
LVH	left ventricular hypertrophy
MHI/ANW	Minneapolis Heart Institute at Abbott Northwestern Hospital
MI	myocardial infarction
MICUs	mobile intensive care units
NCDR	National Cardiovascular Data Registry
NISTE	nonischemic STE
NP	nurse practitioner
NRMI	National Registry of Acute MI
NSTE-ACS	non-ST elevation-acute coronary syndrome
NSTEMI	non-ST-elevation myocardial infarction
OHCA	out-of-hospital cardiac arrest
PCI	percutaneous coronary intervention
PCP	primary care paramedic
PI	pharmacoinvasive
POC	point-of-care
PPCI	primary percutaneous coronary intervention
RBBB	Right bundle branch block
RCTs	randomized controlled trials
REACT	Rapid Early Action for Coronary Treatment
REACT	Rescue Angioplasty versus Conservative Treatment or Repeat Thrombolysis
RIKS-HIA	Register of Information and Knowledge About Swedish Heart Intensive Care Admissions
ROSC	return of spontaneous circulation
SAC	Argentine Cardiology Society
SAMU	Service d'Aide Médicale Urgente
SAR	search and rescue
SRC	STEMI receiving center
STE	ST-segment elevation
STEMI	ST-elevation myocardial infarction
STREAM	Strategic Reperfusion Early After Myocardial Infarction

TIME-NE	Timely Intervention in Myocardial Emergency, North-East
TIMI	Thrombolysis In Myocardial Infarction
TXA2	thromboxane A2
UFH	unfractionated heparin
USIC	Unité de Soins Intensifs Coronaires
VF	ventricular fibrillation
WEST	Which Early ST-elevation MI Therapy
WPW	Wolff-Parkinson-White

INTRODUCTION

Increasing Importance of Prehospital Care of ST-Segment Elevation Myocardial Infarction

Edgardo Escobar, MD, and Alejandro Barbagelata, MD

Due to the emergent nature of acute myocardial infarction (AMI), few events in medicine require such a rapid and coordinated response from our healthcare system. Unfortunately it remains a leading cause of mortality and disability.

Giant steps have been made to abort the ongoing wavefront of myocardial necrosis in AMI with therapies that have dramatically improved clinical outcomes if delivered in a timely manner. Particularly following hospital admission, well established guidelines around the globe allow effective management of AMI.

However, compared to the enormous amount of data available after hospital admission, the prehospital phase of AMI has been mostly overlooked and much less data has been collected and analyzed to determine the optimal management strategy. This results in significant variation of care across different regions.

This is particularly relevant due to the well known early hazard of ST-segment elevation myocardial infarction

Prehospital Management of Acute STEMI: Practical Approaches and International Strategies for Early Intervention © 2015 Joseph S. Alpert, Lynne T. Braun, Barbara J. Fletcher, Gerald Fletcher, Editors-in-Chief, Cardiotext Publishing, ISBN: 978-1-935395-66-9

(STEMI) where most deaths occur before hospital admission. Patients presenting early have a high mortality and get the most benefit from reperfusion therapy. Conversely, those presenting late have already survived the prehospital phase, and are at lower risk of sudden ischemic death and benefit less from reperfusion (the "survivor-cohort effect"). This time related benefit of reperfusion has led to such phrases as "time is muscle" and "time is life"–universal affirmations that the early minutes or hours after AMI onset are indeed the most dangerous. Paradoxically however, management strategies for the prehospital period are not well established and represent a weak link in the chain of AMI management.

Primary percutaneous coronary intervention (PPCI) has become the optimal reperfusion strategy when performed in a timely manner. Since most patients do not present to a PPCI-capable hospital, this factor presents a major logistic challenge in many regions as most centers do not have PPCI capabilities. This situation has created even more pronounced prehospital delays either through travelling longer distances by Emergency Medical Service (EMS) sometimes without having a definite diagnosis or transferring from community hospitals to established centers for PPCI. The end result is delivery of reperfusion therapies outside the guideline recommended times with negative impact on survival.

Over the years both the guidelines and the medical community have focused largely on improving the management of AMI patients following hospital admission, using the metrics of "door-to-balloon" or "door-to-needle" times. A metric that focuses on the time from first contact with the healthcare system to the initiation of reperfusion therapy (system delay) may be more relevant, because this constitutes the total time to reperfusion modifiable by the healthcare system. An even more relevant metric may be the time from symptom onset to treatment referred to as "total ischemic time". Using this metric involves thorough patient education to respond quickly to the onset of symptoms. From this perspective, prompt prehospital diagnosis and treatment of AMI have become increasingly recognized as important determinants of outcome. Diagnosing a STEMI at the earliest possible moment could immediately activate a series of events beginning in the field, leading to more rapid reperfusion and improved survival.

Prehospital diagnosis even by primary care paramedics has been shown to be possible and effective. Acquisition of a 12-lead electrocardiogram by paramedics at the site of first medical contact is recommended in the American College of Cardiology, American Heart Association, and European guidelines. The key trigger point for emergency system activation is usually a single electrocardiogram diagnostic of an acute STEMI. This instantly reclassifies a patient with chest pain from "routine evaluation" to a "high-priority" status and usually initiates an algorithm leading directly to reperfusion therapy, which bypasses community hospitals. In those early presenters with expected long delay for PPCI, a prehospital pharmaco-invasive approach with thrombolytic therapy has also proven to be effective before percutaneous coronary intervention (PCI) is performed.

Improving prehospital care for acute STEMI should encompass a multi-layered approach from multiple levels of the healthcare system including patients, paramedics, nurses, emergency department personnel, cardiologists and policy-makers. Working together in an interprofessional team approach they may not only improve the prehospital phase of AMI management, but also increase the number of AMI patients receiving reperfusion therapy who really need it, while reducing the number of misdiagnoses causing inappropriate or false activations of the health system's AMI algorithm.

Consensus needs to be reached regarding questions that arise every day in practice such as the need for nurses, paramedic and/or physicians to be present at the time of first medical contact, the time to acquire the first 12-lead electrocardiogram and who should interpret it, who should activate the system's AMI algorithm, and when to bypass a community hospital and emergency room. Other questions concern what medications (including thrombolytic therapy) to give en route in non-PPCI covered areas or when significant expected delays in percutaneous coronary intervention (PCI) are anticipated and also the prehospital management of the post-cardiac arrest patient. Finally, newer approaches using wireless technology, such as transmission of the electrocardiogram from the field to an on-call cardiologist or access to an expert that is available at all times via telemedicine, are additional strategies that might be considered to improve and streamline the process.

This book provides an international perspective of the prehospital phase of AMI. Its aims are to emphasize the importance of this phase and share the experience of countries that manage it differently. We hope this effort may help health authorities and cardiology organizations define programs for prehospital AMI care with the goal to achieve optimal reperfusion as early as possible in patients with STEMI. It is our belief that the implementation of well-organized systems of prehospital care will support the goal of saving more lives and prevent unnecessary disability.

Part 1

Program Development for Prehospital STEMI Care Systems: Focus on the United States Experience

CHAPTER 1

Delays and Decision Points in Prehospital STEMI Management Systems: A Framework for Reducing the Gap Between the Scientific Guidelines and the Real-World Experience

Qiangjun Cai, MD, and Alejandro Barbagelata, MD

INTRODUCTION

The total ischemic time during ST elevation myocardial infarction (STEMI) starts as early as the onset of patient symptoms and ends with successful reperfusion of the occluded coronary artery. Prehospital management refers to the interprofessional team and the various components of this total ischemic time. These system components are being evaluated to identify opportunities to improve early identification of STEMI and provide optimal care throughout the entire ischemic time period.

Prehospital Management of Acute STEMI: Practical Approaches and International Strategies for Early Intervention © 2015 Joseph S. Alpert, Lynne T. Braun, Barbara J. Fletcher, Gerald Fletcher, Editors-in-Chief, Cardiotext Publishing, ISBN: 978-1-935395-66-9

For patients transported by emergency medical services (EMS) without a prehospital electrocardiogram (ECG) directly to a hospital with percutaneous coronary intervention (PCI) capabilities, the delay from symptom onset to reperfusion therapy may be divided into these intervals: (1) symptom onset to EMS arrival; (2) EMS arrival to hospital arrival; (3) hospital arrival to ECG; (4) ECG to cardiac catheterization laboratory activation (CLA); and (5) reperfusion. For patients transferred from a referring hospital to a receiving PCI hospital, additional time intervals are added. This chapter examines many of these component intervals and describes current management systems in the United States and other countries.

PATIENT DELAY—EARLY SYMPTOM RECOGNITION

Early STEMI symptom recognition by the patient in order to seek medical attention is critical for survival and muscle salvage. STEMI is responsible for a significant number of deaths related to coronary artery disease, and is the number one cause of death. It comprises approximately 25% to 40% of all acute coronary syndromes.[1] STEMI patients have higher risk during the first few hours after symptom onset ("the early hazard" of STEMI). That explains why a significant number of deaths occur before patients arrive at the hospital.[2] Early presentation and timely reperfusion may abort the ongoing wavefront of myocardial necrosis, thus improving survival and decreasing consequent heart failure.[3]

The American College of Cardiology (ACC)/American Heart Association (AHA) and European Society of Cardiology (ESC) STEMI guidelines describes typical ischemic symptoms or ischemia equivalents.[4–6] The guidelines also recognize that these symptoms are not specific for myocardial ischemia and may be attributed to noncardiac disorders, resulting in misdiagnosis. At least one-third of STEMI patients present with symptoms other than chest pain or even without symptoms. Many patients delay seeking medical attention because they assume that heart attack symptoms should present with severe chest pain.[7]

Patient delay, defined as the time from symptom onset to first medical contact (FMC), postpones potentially life-saving procedures and contributes substantially to a reduced treatment efficacy. The ACC/AHA STEMI guidelines recommend patients call an ambulance if chest pain is unimproved or worsens in 5 minutes.[5,6] However, delayed access to medical care in patients with STEMI is common in the real world. Patients with STEMI do not seek medical care for approximately 1.5 to 4.7 hours after symptom onset.[8,9] Nearly one-third of STEMI patients do not receive early reperfusion therapy, mostly due to late presentation.[10] Barriers to rapid action include insufficient knowledge, poor coping mechanisms, attributing the symptoms to a less serious etiology, and/or embarrassment about being wrong.[11]

Symptom onset is the starting point for the calculation of ischemic time. However, determining the time of symptom onset for STEMI can be challenging. Preceding episodes of unstable angina due to intermittent coronary occlusion often make it difficult to determine the exact moment of symptom onset. And in some cases, ST elevation may not be present on the initial ECG.[12,13] Given the challenges in accurately ascertaining time of symptom onset, various ECG approaches to estimate necrosis/ischemia ratio have been proposed, such as Q-wave development in the area of ST elevation or the acute ischemia index.[14,15]

Few advances have been made in the last 20 years in decreasing this prehospital delay, either because patients do not recognize their symptoms for what they are, or because the first responders are delayed in making the proper diagnosis.[16] The resources and commitment needed to increase early presentation to FMC and to make early diagnoses have been relatively slow in coming. The 20-city Rapid Early Action for

Coronary Treatment (REACT) trial—a randomized, intensive 18-month community-based intervention that targeted mass media, community organizations, and professional, public, and patient education to increase awareness of symptoms of myocardial infarction (MI)—did not improve patient-related delays in seeking medical care.[17,18]

The recently launched AHA's Mission: Lifeline® initiative aims to increase the number of patients with timely access to reperfusion by addressing the continuum of care for STEMI, beginning with patient recognition of symptoms. EMS activation is critical not only for rapid transport to the hospital, but also to provide the opportunity for early assessment and treatment, as well as evaluation of hemodynamic stability, prehospital medical stabilization, prehospital ECG, and expedited communication with the accepting hospital. The 2004 ACC/AHA STEMI guideline recommended patients with symptoms of STEMI be transported to the hospital by ambulance rather than by friends or relatives.[6] Despite this guideline recommendation and its clear benefit during the early, deadly STEMI period, only about 40% to 50% of STEMI patients use EMS.[19] However, since European countries such as Denmark have higher EMS use, and there is a significant variation within the United States, it may be possible to improve EMS use in the United States by identifying and educating the high-risk population, their families, and communities.

SYSTEM DELAY—FIRST MEDICAL CONTACT, DOOR-TO-BALLOON, AND DOOR-IN DOOR-OUT

For patients with STEMI who arrive at a hospital capable of primary percutaneous coronary intervention (PPCI) by private transportation (walk-in), the FMC coincides with door time. However, up to 50% of patients with STEMI in the

United States are transported by EMS.[19] In this latter population, FMC coincides with the time the EMS provider arrives at the patient's side. As only 25% of the US hospitals have PPCI capabilities, the majority of STEMI patients has their FMC either with the EMS unit or with a hospital not capable of PPCI, and so need transfer to a PPCI center. When "walk-in" patients present to a non-PCI center, the FMC is at this referral center, and the event falls within the prehospital phase, relative to the receiving PCI center (Figure 1.1). If the patient is transported by EMS to a non-PCI center, and then again by EMS to a center capable of PCI, then the FMC occurs at the time of the first EMS contact.

The survival benefit of PPCI in STEMI may be reduced if door-to-balloon (D2B) time exceeds door-to-needle time (for fibrinolytic therapy) by one hour.[20] Therefore, both the US and European STEMI guidelines recommend a D2B or FMC to

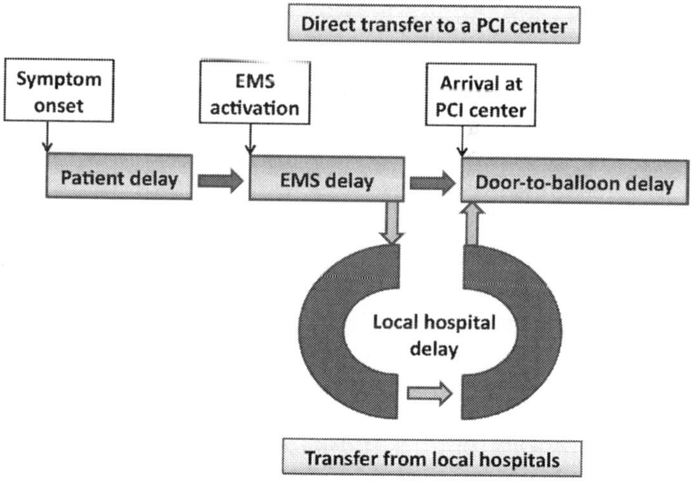

Figure 1.1

Delays in patients with STEMI transported by the emergency medical service.

device time of ≤ 90 minutes, with a maximum door-to-needle time of 30 minutes.[4–6] The Centers for Medicare and Medicaid Services (CMS) and the Joint Commission on Accreditation of Healthcare Organizations used a D2B of 90 minutes as a core measure and in 2005 began reporting hospital D2B times publicly.[21] In 2006, the ACC and 38 partner organizations launched the D2B alliance to improve D2B times.[22,23] The key strategies advocated include cardiac CLA with a single call from the emergency medicine physician, cath team preparation within 20 to 30 minutes of the call, rapid data feedback, a team-based approach, and administrative support. The use of a prehospital ECG by EMS to activate the catheterization laboratory was an optional strategy.[24] The goal of the D2B alliance was 75% of D2B times ≤ 90 minutes.[25] Based on CMS data, D2B time declined from a median of 96 minutes in 2005 to 64 minutes in 2010, with 91.4% of D2B times ≤ 90 minutes.[21] However, although the D2B time may accurately reflect the efficacy of an individual PCI center, it does not take into account overall *system* delays that may include, as mentioned above, all stages between the time of FMC and admission to the PCI center.[2]

Performing PPCI within 90 minutes of FMC is acceptable but not ideal. Better survival strongly correlates with shorter D2B times, indicating that the benefits of PCI increase the sooner it can be done.[26,27] A reduction in D2B time from 90 minutes to 60 minutes was associated with 0.8% lower mortality, and a reduction from 60 minutes to 30 minutes with another 0.5% lower mortality.[26] The most outstanding institutions are now achieving times under 60 minutes through strategies that include coordination with EMS and acquisition of a prehospital ECG.[21] This level of performance may become the new standard. The 2012 ESC STEMI guideline gave a class I recommendation for D2B times of ≤ 60 minutes if the patient presents within 120 minutes of symptom onset, or directly to a hospital capable of PCI.[4] Although the US 2013 guideline still recommends a D2B time of ≤ 90 minutes, it does state that the time to treatment should be as short as possible.

The main problem is that the majority of STEMI patients present to non-PPCI centers, in which case the D2B time stretches from the door of the referring (first) hospital to the balloon of the receiving (second) hospital. In this scenario, D2B delay at the receiving center usually comprises a relatively minor part of the overall (system) delay, with the pre-PCI hospital portion being much longer. In this situation, a curious paradox may arise whereby a shorter receiving center D2B time results from a preceding system delay long enough to allow full preparation at the receiving center. Thus, survival may be worse despite a brief receiving center D2B time.[28] This population remains as a challenge.[28,29] A previous analysis from the National Cardiovascular Data Registry (NCDR) CathPCI Registry showed that less than 10% of transferred patients with STEMI between 2005 and 2007 had an overall D2B time of < 90 minutes.[30] Between 2007 and 2010, the Acute Coronary Treatment and Intervention Outcomes Network (ACTION) Registry—Get With the Guidelines (GWTG) registry showed improvement in overall D2B times for transferred patients with STEMI, with approximately 20% patients treated within an overall D2B time of < 90 minutes.[31]

The 2008 ACC/AHA performance measures for STEMI designated a new performance benchmark, door-in to door-out (DIDO) time, which assesses the amount of time a STEMI patient spends at the referring hospital.[32] The 2013 ACCF/AHA STEMI guideline recommended that DIDO time should not exceed 30 minutes.[5] In the 2007–2010 ACTION-GWTG registry, the median DIDO time was 68 minutes. Patients with a DIDO time of > 30 minutes had increased mortality compared with those treated within 30 minutes (5.9% vs. 2.7%, $P < 0.001$) and were less likely to have an overall D2B time of ≤ 90 minutes.[31] Recently, CMS has considered publicly reporting DIDO times.

Delays in transferring STEMI patients could reduce the survival advantage of PCI enough to favor giving more immediate fibrinolytic therapy at the first (referring) hospital. Among patients with DIDO times >30 minutes, only 0.6% had an absolute contraindication to fibrinolysis, and one study found that transfer PCI conferred no survival advantage over on-site fibrinolysis when total D2B time exceeds 120 minutes.[33] The guidelines recommend D2B times of ≤120 minutes for transfer patients instead of 90 minutes.[5] Based on CMS data, just 9.7% of transfer STEMI patients had DIDO times of ≤30 minutes, and 31.0% had DIDO times of >90 minutes. The median overall D2B time was 120 minutes, and only 19% of transferred patients achieved an overall D2B time of ≤90 minutes.[30]

Long DIDO times most commonly result from various delays within the referring hospital's Emergency Department (ED), and the wait for transport to the receiving PCI hospital.[34] Standardizing transfer protocols, increasing the availability of transport vehicles, and implementing prehospital notification at referring hospitals may lead to earlier dispatching of transport services. ED delay is mainly due to an initially nondiagnostic ECG, which is best addressed by obtaining serial ECGs.[34]

Even though >50% of STEMI patients have their FMC with EMS, the subsequent system delays of this situation have been difficult to address. Linking prehospital EMS data with in-hospital STEMI data may provide more insight into system-related delay. Such data analysis of the North Carolina STEMI Registry demonstrated that for those transported directly to a PCI center, 53% reached the 90-minutes target guideline goal. For those transferred from a non-PCI facility, only 24% reached the 120-minutes target goal for PPCI.[35]

PREHOSPITAL ECG

The 2004 ACC/AHA STEMI guideline stated that it is reasonable to perform a 12-lead ECG routinely on chest-pain patients suspected of STEMI (class IIa recommendation).[6] The newly published 2013 ACCF/AHA STEMI guideline has upgraded this recommendation to class I, requiring EMS to obtain a 12-lead ECG at the site of FMC.[5] This is consistent with the 2012 ESC STEMI guideline stating that a 12-lead ECG must be obtained as soon as possible at the point of FMC, with a target delay of ≤10 minutes (class I).

Timely acquisition of a prehospital ECG upon FMC by EMS represents an evidence-based strategy to reduce reperfusion time in STEMI patients.[36–39] A pooled analysis of 10 registries showed that 86% of STEMI patients diagnosed by a prehospital ECG and transported directly to a PPCI center had a D2B time of <90 minutes, and each individual registry surpassed the ACC D2B alliance benchmark of 75% of STEMI patients with acceptable D2B times.[39] A recent study from Denmark suggested that with a prehospital ECG diagnosis and direct referral for PPCI, the system delays of STEMI patients living far from a PCI center are comparable to those living close by.[38] A properly diagnosed prehospital ECG for STEMI patients reduced both scene and transport time, and so reduced total ischemic time.[37]

For patients transported by EMS without a prehospital ECG, the delay from symptom onset to reperfusion therapy may be divided into these intervals: (1) symptom onset to EMS arrival; (2) EMS arrival to hospital arrival; (3) hospital arrival to ECG; and (4) ECG to reperfusion. For patients transferred from a referring hospital to a receiving PCI hospital, one must add (5) DIDO time; (6) transfer to the receiving hospital; and (7) receiving hospital D2B time. If prehospital ECG programs were effectively implemented and coordinated with hospital systems, intervals (2)–(4) might decrease. Interval (4) could be decreased by notifying the hospital to activate the catheterization laboratory while the patient is still en route. A prehospital ECG could decrease DIDO times and eventually allow EMS units to bypass non-PCI hospitals.

However, despite these guidelines and the availability of EMS equipment in 200 major cities, the use of prehospital ECGs to diagnose and facilitate the treatment of STEMI remains low in the United States.[40] Data from the NCDR ACTION registry showed that EMS units obtained prehospital ECGs on just 27% of STEMI patients.[41] Several barriers slow the implementation of prehospital 12-lead ECG programs. They require equipment, paramedic training, and repeated assessments of paramedic competency. There is a lack of well-designed clinical studies assessing the cost-effectiveness of acquiring, interpreting, and transmitting prehospital ECGs. In addition, using prehospital ECGs will likely steer at least some STEMI patients away from community hospitals, and thus adversely affect their financial standing.

The central challenge for healthcare providers is not simply to perform a prehospital ECG, but to appropriately declare a medical emergency by timely and accurate interpretation of the tracing, and to integrate the prehospital ECG findings with the broader systems of care. Although the STEMI guidelines do not specify who should interpret ECG and triage the patient, if done improperly, these steps may result in either false system activation or delayed patient reperfusion and could prompt litigious action, especially if the patient is harmed by the decisions of an unaccredited individual.

Various methods of ECG interpretation have been proposed: (1) using a computer algorithm (Los Angeles, CA)[39]; (2) paramedic interpretation (Boston, MA)[42]; (3) physician interpretation via wireless or fax transmission,[43] (4) online feedback via telemedicine from an experienced cardiologist available at all times (South America); and (5) interpretation by a physicians/cardiologist on board the EMS unit (European).[43,44] Part 2 of this book contains chapters from several countries in South America and Europe describing these ECG systems and their impact on prehospital STEMI management. EMS units in the United States are staffed by paramedics, and physicians must rely on computer-assisted or paramedic ECG interpretations that may increase the number of false-positive and -negative STEMI diagnoses.[36] Because the highest mortality of STEMI occurs within the first few hours, efforts and resources should be aimed at using the most capable personnel to acquire and properly interpret the ECG as soon as possible.

FALSE ACTIVATION—THE "COLLATERAL DAMAGE" OF REDUCING TIME TO REPERFUSION

Early identification of STEMI, especially in the prehospital setting, and rapid activation of a cardiac catheterization laboratory have reduced the morbidity and mortality of STEMI patients by decreasing their total ischemic and D2B times. But frequently the catheterization laboratory must be activated despite inconclusive incoming data, and is found in retrospect to have been unnecessary. Thus, the pressure to expedite STEMI care may produce "collateral damage" in the form of false system activation, when presumed STEMI patients are ultimately found to not require emergent coronary angiography or do not have a coronary occlusion.[45] The D2B alliance emphasizes using methods shown to reduce D2B time as a core quality measure of PPCI. Although the STEMI guidelines do not specifically recommend how or by whom the catheterization laboratory should be activated, they endorse the strategies of the D2B alliance.[4–6] Hospitals involved in the alliance follow recommendations to expedite care by allowing EMS personnel or Emergency Department physicians to activate the catheterization laboratory without cardiology consultation.[46] The gains of this strategy must be weighed against the drawback of unnecessary CLAs.

The prevalence of false-positive CLA varies from 5% to 36%, depending on who initiates the activation and the definitions used.[47–50] In a registry of 1335 patients with suspected STEMI whose angiographies were requested by ED physicians, 14% had no culprit lesion and 9.5% had no significant coronary artery disease.[51] Among 3973 activations in a state-wide North Carolina program, 15% were inappropriate. The rate of cancellation because of reinterpretation of ECG was 6% for all EMS activations and 4.6% for ED physicians.[52] McCabe et al. reported a 36% incidence of false-positive activations by ED physicians. Among these, 12.8% were because of mistaken ECG interpretation. In contrast, only 82% of patients with ST-elevation on their initial ECG received a final diagnosis of STEMI.[47]

Unnecessary emergent coronary angiography is not without risk to the patient and may burden limited catheterization laboratory resources. Measurable costs include emergency transportation, laboratory personnel, equipment, and other materials. Less tangible costs include the exposure of patients to the risks and possible complications of unnecessary angiography. Repeated unnecessary activation may also weaken regional STEMI collaborations ("STEMI fatigue") if catheterization laboratory staff become reluctant to respond to emergency physicians or paramedics who "cry wolf" too often. This could blunt their responsiveness to any future STEMI activations.

The different definitions and terms for "false activation" reflect its various causes. The Mission: Lifeline program accepts phrases such as "protocol deviation" or "lab cancellation." Activations may prove incorrect because an ECG is misinterpreted, or because the ECG is interpreted correctly, yet the patient still does not have a STEMI (Figure 1.2). An appropriate but false-positive activation is defined as the absence of a total or subtotal thrombotic coronary occlusion despite the ECG meeting STEMI guideline class I criteria for activation. Although STEMI guidelines have explicit voltage criteria defining ST elevation, they also acknowledge that many conditions such as acute pericarditis, left ventricular hypertrophy,

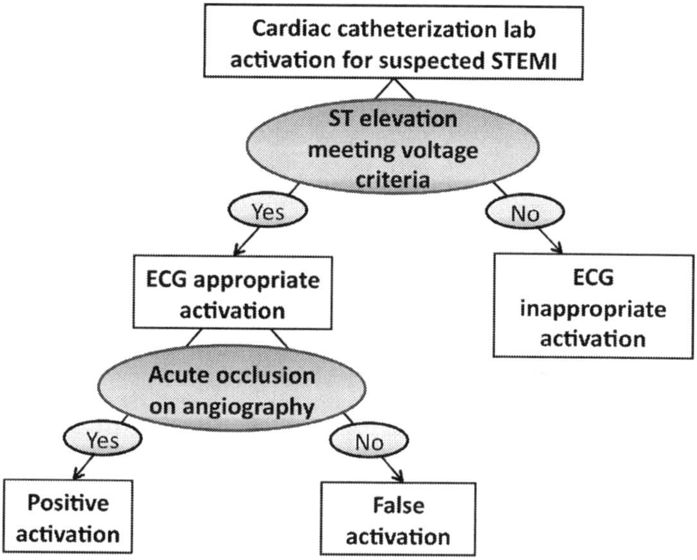

Figure 1.2

Classification scheme for evaluation of CLAs.

early repolarization, and left bundle branch block (LBBB) can mimic the ST elevation caused by a STEMI.[48,53] In general, the guidelines favor declaring an emergency over denying reperfusion, knowing that an estimated 30% of STEMI patients are not reperfused in a timely manner.[54] This critical decision-making process must balance the sensitivity in detecting all potential candidates who may benefit from reperfusion against the specificity of system activation and resource utilization. The quality of acute reperfusion therapy should be judged not only by door-to-treatment times but also by the ratio of appropriate to inappropriate activation of reperfusion therapy.

The 2004 ACC/AHA and 2012 ESC STEMI guidelines regard chest pain with a new or presumably new LBBB an STEMI equivalent and a class I indication for emergent reperfusion therapy.[4,6] However, accumulating angiographic evidence suggests that this is a frequent cause of false cardiac cath lab activation.[55–57] Using the Sgarbossa ECG criteria is a well-validated method for diagnosing a STEMI in the presence of LBBB. A Sgarbossa score of ≥ 3 has a superb specificity (98%) and positive predictive value for acute MI and angiography-confirmed acute coronary occlusion. The newly published 2013 STEMI guideline recognizes that most cases of LBBB at time of presentation are "not known to be old" because an ECG obtained previous to the event is not available for comparison. Physicians must make prompt decisions and have little time to interpret complex ECGs or determine whether a LBBB is new or old. The new guideline has removed its previous recommendations regarding LBBB.[5] This change from "all comers" to "none" with LBBB will no doubt reduce the number of false CLAs. However, as with any increase in specificity, the accompanying loss of sensitivity will result in delaying the reperfusion of some patients who truly have a STEMI, which could be fatal. Thus, a new diagnosis and triage algorithm incorporating the Sgarbossa and modified Sgarbossa ECG criteria has been proposed.[58,59]

SYSTEMS OF CARE—THE AHA MISSION: LIFELINE® PROGRAM STEMI NETWORKS

Although PPCI is the most effective reperfusion therapy for STEMI if timely delivered,[60] a significant number of STEMI patients do not undergo PCI when it is the only reperfusion option.[61] Major improvements in STEMI outcomes are possible if systems of care are developed that can coordinate and integrate all phases of treatment, including prehospital events, community hospitals not capable of PCI, EDs, and cardiology services.[62] The AHA Mission: Lifeline initiative is part of the national effort to regionalize STEMI care. This program focuses on each component of STEMI systems of care to improve regional access to PPCI and reduce the time to reperfusion. The 2013 ACCF/AHA STEMI guideline recommends as class I the creation and maintenance of regional systems of STEMI care that include the assessment and continuous quality improvement of EMS and hospital-based activities.[5] It states that system development can be facilitated by participating in programs such as Mission: Lifeline. The European equivalent to Mission: Lifeline is Stent for Life, tailored to help specific national healthcare settings improve access to timely and effective PPCI through focused implementation programs.[63]

The D2B time is an important parameter for monitoring the quality of care within PPCI centers, but it does not reflect all components of the healthcare system that may be improved when treating STEMI patients. System delay (the interval from the first alert of the healthcare system to the initiation of reperfusion therapy) might be a better performance measure, because it incorporates the time required for each step of therapy and, if reduced, would further improve the mortality and decrease the incidence of heart failure in STEMI patients undergoing PPCI.[2,64] A strategy of prehospital diagnosis and rerouting patients directly to a catheterization laboratory may shorten system delay by as much as one hour. D2B time may of course continue as one measure of PCI center performance.

The 2013 ACCF/AHA STEMI guideline recommends as class I that EMS transport STEMI patients directly to a PCI-capable hospital for PPCI.[5] Traditionally, the majority of community protocols instruct EMS units to transport chest-pain patients to the nearest hospital, even if that hospital cannot provide PPCI. The reasons include patient preference and preventing a negative perception of the bypassed hospital that might affect its finances. However, the guidelines recognize that, compared to those patients referred from the EDs of non-PCI hospitals, acceptable FMC-to-balloon times are more often achieved if trained paramedics independently triage patients and bypass non-PCI hospitals if necessary (79.7 vs. 11.9%).[28,65–67] This strategy is also associated with a significant reduction in mortality, heart failure, and cardiogenic shock compared to those patients referred from a non-PCI hospital.[68,69] Therefore, regions should develop STEMI systems that incorporate standardized protocols to facilitate rapid transfer of STEMI patients. The model mirrors existing US trauma systems, which identify high-risk patients in the field and transport them directly to a hospital designated as best equipped and staffed to deal with that situation. The system in Boston is a good example of one that allows paramedics to bypass non-PCI-capable hospitals when a STEMI patient has been identified in the field.

The development of regional STEMI receiving center (SRC) networks is another key means of improving accessibility to PCI for STEMI patients who present first to a non-PCI hospital. Large clinical trials and registries show that well-organized interfacility transfer of PCI patients to tertiary care centers is superior to giving fibrinolytic therapy at the initial, non-PCI hospital. A meta-analysis of 6 randomized clinical trials (3750 patients) that compared these 2 strategies showed that the combined endpoint of death, reinfarction, and stroke at 30 days was less by 42% in the patients expeditiously transferred to a PCI center compared to a group receiving fibrinolytic therapy. Thus, transfer for PCI appears feasible, safe, and worth the wait when using such systems. One of the first SRC networks was established in 2003 in Minneapolis, MN, where a hub-and-spoke system was developed between Abbott Northwestern Hospital, the designated SRC, and a number of hospitals within a 200-mile radius.[70] A standardized protocol has been implemented successfully in 30 rural and community hospitals. Door-to-balloon times of ≤ 120 minutes were achieved in 79% and 49% of patients located < 60 and 60 to 210 miles away, respectively. By comparison, the National Registry of Myocardial Infarction concurrently reported that 16% of transferred patients and 65% of patients at PCI hospitals achieved times of < 120 minutes. The Abbott Northwestern Hospital SRC triage system and protocols are described more fully in Chapter 5: *Triage Models for ST-Elevation Myocardial Infarction Systems of Prehospital Care and the Challenge of Inappropriate Cardiac Catheterization Laboratory Activation.*

Improving systems of care for STEMI patients requires a multifaceted approach that includes patient education, engaging the EMS and EDs of both the referral and receiving centers, and encouraging advocacy groups to work with payers and policy makers in redesigning these components of the healthcare system. At the very least, improvements in EMS utilization and the accurate and timely reading of a prehospital ECG will be necessary. Interactions between EMS providers and hospitals are critical if STEMI systems of care are to be successful.[19] If done improperly, costs may increase without clinical benefit.

CARDIAC ARREST IN STEMI—TIME IS LIFE: EXTENDING THE CHAIN OF SURVIVAL

Acute ischemic events cause most out-of-hospital cardiac arrests (OHCA) that occur without an extracardiac etiology. Although the 2004 ACC/AHA STEMI guideline has no explicit recommendations regarding the invasive evaluation of OHCA patients,[6] both the 2013 ACCF/AHA and the 2012 ESC STEMI guidelines,[4,5] and the AHA 2010 guideline for cardiopulmonary resuscitation and emergency cardiovascular care[71] give a class I recommendation for performing immediate angiography and PCI if a resuscitated OHCA patient's initial ECG shows STEMI. In addition, the 2012 ESC STEMI guideline recommends (class IIa) immediate angiography and PCI in survivors of cardiac arrest if their ECG lacks diagnostic ECG ST elevation, but there is other strong evidence for acute infarction, such as a report of chest pain immediately preceding the arrest, an established history of coronary atherosclerosis, and abnormal or uncertain ECG findings.[4]

Routinely using such invasive strategies on all postresuscitation patients presenting without ST elevation is a matter of debate. The absence of ST elevation on a postresuscitation ECG may not rule out an ischemic event, and early angiography might be necessary for a diagnosis. In the Parisian Region Out-of-Hospital Cardiac Arrest Registry, a coronary angiogram was routinely performed in patients with no obvious noncardiac cause of arrest regardless of clinical and ECG findings. Significant coronary artery stenosis was found in 96% of patients with ST elevation and in 58% of patients without ST elevation on the postresuscitation ECG. The hospital survival rate was 31% in patients with no or failed PCI and 51% in those successfully revascularized. The negative predictive value of ST elevation for coronary artery occlusion was only 0.42. These data strongly suggest that anyone successfully resuscitated from OHCA thought to be cardiac in origin should undergo emergent coronary angiography, regardless of their postresuscitation ECG findings.[72]

Whether emergent coronary angiography and PCI should be performed on postarrest patients that remain unconscious at the time of the procedure is part of this debate. Although the interventionalist might avoid these patients because of their presumably bad effect on publicly reported outcomes, some have claimed that a patient's immediate postresuscitation neurological function, even if comatose, should not affect the decision to perform emergent coronary angiography and PCI.[73,74] Gorjup et al. reported that STEMI patients who were successfully resuscitated from OHCA but remained comatose at the time of catheterization still had a survival-to-hospital discharge rate of 51%, and the hospital survival with cerebral performance category 1 or 2 was 29%.[75]

The concept of a system of care also applies to STEMI patients suffering cardiac arrest. Prompt recognition of symptoms, bystander life support, a properly diagnosed prehospital ECG, appropriate activation of remaining system components, and EMS transport for early angiography and hypothermia are all of paramount importance. As for STEMI occurring without collapse, the AHA has issued a policy statement calling for communities to establish regional systems of care for OHCA.[76] PCI-capable hospitals become the ideal candidates to serve as Level I cardiac resuscitation centers.[77] For detailed discussion, please consult Chapter 6: *Prehospital STEMI Management in the Setting of Out-of-Hospital Cardiac Arrest.*

PREHOSPITAL FIBRINOLYSIS OR PHARMACOINVASIVE THERAPY IN THE REAL WORLD—WHY IT DOES NOT WORK IN THE UNITED STATES

Randomized trials comparing fibrinolytic therapy to PPCI for treatment of STEMI have consistently shown that the interventional approach is superior.[78] However, the majority of STEMI patients who present to non-PCI facilities do not undergo PPCI within guideline-recommended times. Recent data from Denmark and the United States show that the total D2B times for 65% to 80% of STEMI patients transferred from non-PCI centers remains > 120 minutes.[79] In addition, up to one-third of eligible STEMI patients in the industrialized countries do not receive either form of reperfusion therapy.[61] The appropriate and timely use of some reperfusion therapy is more beneficial than giving none.

The 2012 ESC STEMI guideline recommends as class IIa fibrinolytic therapy for patients presenting < 2 hours after symptom onset who have a large infarct, a low bleeding risk, and an anticipated FMC-to-balloon time of >90 minutes.[4] If possible, fibrinolysis should start in the prehospital setting. Prehospital fibrinolytic therapy is recommended as class IIa in the 2004 ACC/AHA STEMI guideline but is not specified in the 2013 guideline.[5,6] A meta-analysis of 6 randomized trials (6434 patients) showed that prehospital fibrinolysis decreased all-cause mortality by 17% when compared to patient groups receiving in-hospital fibrinolysis.[80,81] These data suggest that fibrinolytic agents given in non-PCI hospitals might be regarded as "prehospital treatment," relative to PPCI centers.

Prehospital fibrinolysis is seldom administered in the United States despite its known benefits and the country's large rural population. There are a number of reasons for this. Since PPCI is accepted as the default reperfusion strategy, both the guidelines and the community have focused on the D2B metric. A successful prehospital fibrinolysis program requires a complex and well-coordinated prehospital system for the prompt and accurate recognition and skilled management of a STEMI. Ideally, there should be a physician in the ambulance, or one that the paramedics can easily consult at any time. Emergency physicians may be reluctant to authorize prehospital fibrinolysis for patients they have not evaluated in person, for fear of litigation. However, about 40% of prehospital fibrinolytic therapy is administered by nonphysician providers.[82] The effectiveness and safety of prehospital fibrinolysis was not influenced by the presence of a physician as demonstrated in the ASSENT 3 PLUS and ER-TIMI-23 trials, and real-world registries.[80,83,84] Another challenge is the regional variation of EMS resources. EMS systems in the United States are particularly fractionated with respect to their funding and available services. For example, rural America—with its long distances and paucity of PCI centers—could be the ideal location for a prehospital fibrinolytic system, yet EMS resources are especially scarce in these areas.[85]

An ECG is a prerequisite for prehospital fibrinolysis. However, only a minority of US prehospital medical services can perform ECGs and transmit them from their ambulances. And even if a computer or paramedic can interpret the ECG in the ambulance, this increases the likelihood of rendering a false positive diagnosis, resulting in unnecessary STEMI treatment and its attendant liability, making providers hesitant.[86] This potential barrier to efficient STEMI management is described fully in Chapter 3: *Prehospital ECG Acquisition/Interpretation: Emerging Technology Applied to STEMI Care.*

Recent clinical trials suggest that a "pharmacoinvasive" strategy coupling early fibrinolysis with routine early invasive management (PCI if warranted), when used early after the onset of symptoms, produces outcomes similar to those achieved by direct PCI.[82,87] In a combined analysis of 1168 STEMI patients from the CAPTIM and WEST trials, the 1-year mortality of patients receiving prehospital fibrinolysis was not statistically different from those receiving direct PCI (4.6% vs. 6.5%, $P = 0.263$). The benefit of prehospital fibrinolytic therapy was demonstrable when delivered within 2 hours of symptom onset.[88] In STEMI patients treated within 2 hours of symptom onset, the CAPTIM trial demonstrated a 5-year mortality of 5.8% in the prehospital fibrinolysis group, and 11.1% in the primary angioplasty group.[89,90] Comparing this reperfusion strategy with PPCI, the recently published STREAM trial found that the outcomes (death, shock, congestive heart failure, or reinfarction up to 30 days) in STEMI patients presenting within 3 hours of symptom onset were similar and there was no significantly increased risk of intracranial bleeding.[91] This combined reperfusion strategy has been implemented in large regional STEMI systems in the United States, such as the Minneapolis Heart Institute's Level 1 MI program and the Mayo Clinic STEMI system.[85] With different but effective reperfusion strategies available, the physician might tailor therapy to fit a particular STEMI patient.[79] Figure 1.3 is one example of a

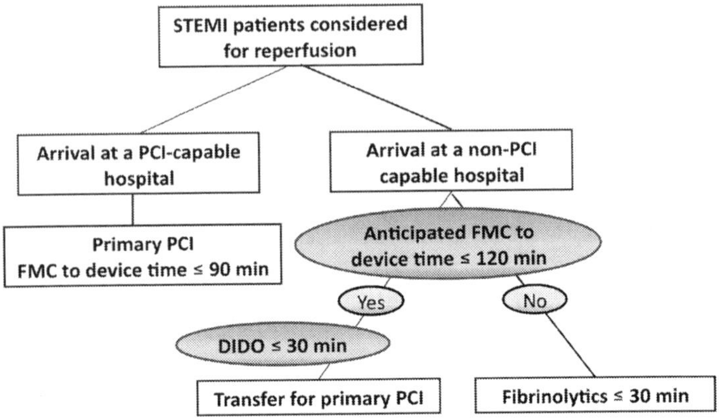

Figure 1.3

Reperfusion therapy for patients with STEMI.

schematic for tailored reperfusion therapy based on different times of presentation after symptom onset.

CONCLUSION

Systems of prehospital STEMI care involve interdependent networks of technology, transportation, communication, and an interprofessional team of personnel. The next chapters describe these system components in more detail. The optimal organization in various countries will vary based on the regional demographics and resources. Additional examples of care systems from different countries are presented to demonstrate a variety of approaches to these systems of care and encourage ongoing collaboration for program development.

REFERENCES

1. Roger VL, Go AS, Lloyd-Jones DM, et al. Executive summary: heart disease and stroke statistics – 2012 update: a report from the American Heart Association. *Circulation*. 2012;125(1):188–197.

2. Terkelsen CJ, Sorensen JT, Maeng M, et al. System delay and mortality among patients with STEMI treated with primary percutaneous coronary intervention. *JAMA.* 2010;304(7):763–771.
3. Terkelsen CJ, Jensen LO, Tilsted HH, et al. Health care system delay and heart failure in patients with ST-segment elevation myocardial infarction treated with primary percutaneous coronary intervention: follow-up of population-based medical registry data. *Ann Intern Med.* 2011;155(6):361–367.
4. Steg PG, James SK, Atar D, et al. ESC Guidelines for the management of acute myocardial infarction in patients presenting with ST-segment elevation. *Eur Heart J.* 2012;33(20):2569–2619.
5. O'Gara PT, Kushner FG, Ascheim DD, et al. 2013 ACCF/AHA guideline for the management of ST-elevation myocardial infarction: a report of the American College of Cardiology Foundation/American Heart Association Task Force on Practice Guidelines. *Circulation.* 2013;127(4):e362–e425.
6. Antman EM, Anbe DT, Armstrong PW, et al. ACC/AHA guidelines for the management of patients with ST-elevation myocardial infarction; A report of the American College of Cardiology/American Heart Association Task Force on Practice Guidelines (Committee to Revise the 1999 Guidelines for the Management of patients with acute myocardial infarction). *J Am Coll Cardiol.* 2004;44(3):E1–E211.
7. Brieger D, Eagle KA, Goodman SG, et al. Acute coronary syndromes without chest pain, an underdiagnosed and undertreated high-risk group: Insights from the Global Registry of Acute Coronary Events. *Chest.* 2004;126(2):461–469.
8. Goldberg RJ, Spencer FA, Fox KA, et al. Prehospital delay in patients with acute coronary syndromes (from the Global Registry of Acute Coronary Events [GRACE]). *Am J Cardiol.* 2009;103(5):598–603.
9. Goldberg RJ, Steg PG, Sadiq I, et al. Extent of, and factors associated with, delay to hospital presentation in patients with acute coronary disease (the GRACE registry). *Am J Cardiol.* 2002;89(7):791–796.
10. Eagle KA, Goodman SG, Avezum A, et al. Practice variation and missed opportunities for reperfusion in ST-segment-elevation myocardial infarction: Findings from the Global Registry of Acute Coronary Events (GRACE). *Lancet.* 2002;359(9304):373–377.
11. Luepker RV. Barriers to patients seeking emergency care for acute coronary heart disease. *JAMA.* 2000;284(17):2184.
12. Riley RF, Newby LK, Don CW, et al. Diagnostic time course, treatment, and in-hospital outcomes for patients with ST-segment elevation myocardial infarction presenting with nondiagnostic initial electrocardiogram: A report from the American Heart Association Mission: Lifeline program. *Am Heart J.* 2013;165(1):50–56.
13. Hackett D, Davies G, Chierchia S, Maseri A. Intermittent coronary occlusion in acute myocardial infarction. Value of

combined thrombolytic and vasodilator therapy. *N Engl J Med.* 1987;317(17):1055–1059.

14. Armstrong PW, Fu Y, Westerhout CM, et al. Baseline Q-wave surpasses time from symptom onset as a prognostic marker in ST-segment elevation myocardial infarction patients treated with primary percutaneous coronary intervention. *J Am Coll Cardiol.* 2009;53(17):1503–1509.
15. Engblom H, Strauss DG, Heden B, et al. The evaluation of an electrocardiographic myocardial ischemia acuteness score to predict the amount of myocardial salvage achieved by early percutaneous coronary intervention clinical validation with myocardial perfusion single photon emission computed tomography and cardiac magnetic resonance. *J Electrocardiol.* 2011;44(5):525–532.
16. Barbagelata A, Perna ER, Clemmensen P, et al. Time to reperfusion in acute myocardial infarction. It is time to reduce it! *J Electrocardiol.* 2007;40(3):257–264.
17. Goff DC, Jr., Feldman HA, McGovern PG, et al. Prehospital delay in patients hospitalized with heart attack symptoms in the United States: the REACT trial. Rapid Early Action for Coronary Treatment (REACT) Study Group. *Am Heart J.* 1999;138(6 Pt 1):1046–1057.
18. Luepker RV, Raczynski JM, Osganian S, et al. Effect of a community intervention on patient delay and emergency medical service use in acute coronary heart disease: the Rapid Early Action for Coronary Treatment (REACT) Trial. *JAMA.* 2000;284(1):60–67.
19. Mathews R, Peterson ED, Li S, et al. Use of emergency medical service transport among patients with ST-segment-elevation myocardial infarction: findings from the National Cardiovascular Data Registry Acute Coronary Treatment Intervention Outcomes Network Registry-Get With The Guidelines. *Circulation.* 2011;124(2):154–163.
20. Pinto DS, Kirtane AJ, Nallamothu BK, et al. Hospital delays in reperfusion for ST-elevation myocardial infarction: implications when selecting a reperfusion strategy. *Circulation.* 2006;114(19):2019–2025.
21. Krumholz HM, Herrin J, Miller LE, et al. Improvements in door-to-balloon time in the United States, 2005 to 2010. *Circulation.* 2011;124(9):1038–1045.
22. Bradley EH, Roumanis SA, Radford MJ, et al. Achieving door-to-balloon times that meet quality guidelines: how do successful hospitals do it? *J Am Coll Cardiol.* 2005;46(7):1236–1241.
23. Krumholz HM, Bradley EH, Nallamothu BK, et al. A campaign to improve the timeliness of primary percutaneous coronary intervention: Door-to-Balloon: An Alliance for Quality. *JACC Cardiovasc Interv.* 2008;1(1):97–104.
24. Bradley EH, Herrin J, Wang Y, et al. Strategies for reducing the door-to-balloon time in acute myocardial infarction. *N Engl J Med.* 2006;355(22):2308–2320.

25. Bradley EH, Nallamothu BK, Herrin J, et al. National efforts to improve door-to-balloon time results from the Door-to-Balloon Alliance. *J Am Coll Cardiol.* 2009;54(25):2423–2429.
26. Rathore SS, Curtis JP, Chen J, et al. Association of door-to-balloon time and mortality in patients admitted to hospital with ST elevation myocardial infarction: national cohort study. *BMJ.* 2009;338:b1807.
27. McNamara RL, Wang Y, Herrin J, et al. Effect of door-to-balloon time on mortality in patients with ST-segment elevation myocardial infarction. *J Am Coll Cardiol.* 2006;47(11):2180–2186.
28. Wang TY, Peterson ED, Ou FS, et al. Door-to-balloon times for patients with ST-segment elevation myocardial infarction requiring interhospital transfer for primary percutaneous coronary intervention: a report from the national cardiovascular data registry. *Am Heart J.* 2011;161(1):76–83.e71.
29. Boden WE, Eagle K, Granger CB. Reperfusion strategies in acute ST-segment elevation myocardial infarction: a comprehensive review of contemporary management options. *J Am Coll Cardiol.* 2007;50(10):917–929.
30. Herrin J, Miller LE, Turkmani DF, et al. National performance on door-in to door-out time among patients transferred for primary percutaneous coronary intervention. *Arch Intern Med.* 2011;171(21):1879–1886.
31. Wang TY, Nallamothu BK, Krumholz HM, et al. Association of door-in to door-out time with reperfusion delays and outcomes among patients transferred for primary percutaneous coronary intervention. *JAMA.* 2011;305(24):2540–2547.
32. Krumholz HM, Anderson JL, Bachelder BL, et al. ACC/AHA 2008 performance measures for adults with ST-elevation and non-ST-elevation myocardial infarction: a report of the American College of Cardiology/American Heart Association Task Force on Performance Measures (Writing Committee to develop performance measures for ST-elevation and non-ST-elevation myocardial infarction): developed in collaboration with the American Academy of Family Physicians and the American College of Emergency Physicians: endorsed by the American Association of Cardiovascular and Pulmonary Rehabilitation, Society for Cardiovascular Angiography and Interventions, and Society of Hospital Medicine. *Circulation.* 2008;118(24):2596–2648.
33. Pinto DS, Frederick PD, Chakrabarti AK, et al. Benefit of transferring ST-segment-elevation myocardial infarction patients for percutaneous coronary intervention compared with administration of onsite fibrinolytic declines as delays increase. *Circulation.* 2011;124(23):2512–2521.
34. Miedema MD, Newell MC, Duval S, et al. Causes of delay and associated mortality in patients transferred with ST-segment-elevation myocardial infarction. *Circulation.* 2011;124(15):1636–1644.

35. Fosbol EL, Granger CB, Peterson ED, et al. Prehospital system delay in ST-segment elevation myocardial infarction care: a novel linkage of emergency medicine services and in hospital registry data. *Am Heart J.* 2013;165(3):363–370.
36. Ting HH, Krumholz HM, Bradley EH, et al. Implementation and integration of prehospital ECGs into systems of care for acute coronary syndrome: A scientific statement from the American Heart Association Interdisciplinary Council on Quality of Care and Outcomes Research, Emergency Cardiovascular Care Committee, Council on Cardiovascular Nursing, and Council on Clinical Cardiology. *Circulation.* 2008;118(10):1066–1079.
37. Patel M, Dunford JV, Aguilar S, et al. Pre-hospital electrocardiography by emergency medical personnel: Effects on scene and transport times for chest pain and ST-segment elevation myocardial infarction patients. *J Am Coll Cardiol.* 2012;60(9):806–811.
38. Sorensen JT, Terkelsen CJ, Norgaard BL, et al. Urban and rural implementation of pre-hospital diagnosis and direct referral for primary percutaneous coronary intervention in patients with acute ST-elevation myocardial infarction. *Eur Heart J.* 2011;32(4):430–436.
39. Rokos IC, French WJ, Koenig WJ, et al. Integration of pre-hospital electrocardiograms and ST-elevation myocardial infarction receiving center (SRC) networks: Impact on Door-to-Balloon times across 10 independent regions. *JACC Cardiovasc Interv.* 2009;2(4):339–346.
40. Williams DM. 2006 JEMS 200-city survey. EMS from all angles. *JEMS.* 2007;32(2):38–42, 44, 46 passim.
41. Diercks DB, Kontos MC, Chen AY, et al. Utilization and impact of pre-hospital electrocardiograms for patients with acute ST-segment elevation myocardial infarction: Data from the NCDR (National Cardiovascular Data Registry) ACTION (Acute Coronary Treatment and Intervention Outcomes Network) Registry. *J Am Coll Cardiol.* 2009;53(2):161–166.
42. Daudelin DH, Sayah AJ, Kwong M, et al. Improving use of prehospital 12-lead ECG for early identification and treatment of acute coronary syndrome and ST-elevation myocardial infarction. *Circ Cardiovasc Qual Outcomes.* 2010;3(3):316–323.
43. Clark EN, Sejersten M, Clemmensen P, Macfarlane PW. Automated electrocardiogram interpretation programs versus cardiologists' triage decision making based on teletransmitted data in patients with suspected acute coronary syndrome. *Am J Cardiol.* 2010;106(12):1696–1702.
44. Campbell PT, Patterson J, Cromer D, et al. Prehospital triage of acute myocardial infarction: wireless transmission of electrocardiograms to the on-call cardiologist via a handheld computer. *J Electrocardiol.* 2005;38(4):300–309.

45. Barbagelata A, Ware DL. Denying reperfusion or falsely declaring emergency: The dilemma posed by ST-segment elevation. *J Electrocardiol.* 2006;39(4 suppl.):S73–S74.
46. Bradley EH, Herrin J, Wang Y, et al. Door-to-drug and door-to-balloon times: where can we improve? Time to reperfusion therapy in patients with ST-segment elevation myocardial infarction (STEMI). *Am Heart J.* 2006;151(6):1281–1287.
47. McCabe JM, Armstrong EJ, Kulkarni A, et al. Prevalence and factors associated with false-positive ST-segment elevation myocardial infarction diagnoses at primary percutaneous coronary intervention-capable centers: a report from the Activate-SF registry. *Arch Intern Med.* 2012;172(11):864–871.
48. Rokos IC, French WJ, Mattu A, et al. Appropriate cardiac cath lab activation: optimizing electrocardiogram interpretation and clinical decision-making for acute ST-elevation myocardial infarction. *Am Heart J.* 2010;160(6):995–1003.e1–8.
49. Kontos MC, Kurz MC, Roberts CS, et al. An evaluation of the accuracy of emergency physician activation of the cardiac catheterization laboratory for patients with suspected ST-segment elevation myocardial infarction. *Ann Emerg Med.* 2010;55(5):423–430.
50. Lee CH, Van Gelder CM, Cone DC. Early cardiac catheterization laboratory activation by paramedics for patients with ST-segment elevation myocardial infarction on prehospital 12-lead electrocardiograms. *Prehosp Emerg Care.* 2010;14(2):153–158.
51. Larson DM, Menssen KM, Sharkey SW, et al. "False-positive" cardiac catheterization laboratory activation among patients with suspected ST-segment elevation myocardial infarction. *JAMA.* 2007;298(23):2754–2760.
52. Garvey JL, Monk L, Granger CB, et al. Rates of cardiac catheterization cancelation for ST-segment elevation myocardial infarction after activation by emergency medical services or emergency physicians: results from the North Carolina Catheterization Laboratory Activation Registry. *Circulation.* 2012;125(2):308–313.
53. Thygesen K, Alpert JS, Jaffe AS, et al. Third universal definition of myocardial infarction. *Circulation.* 2012;126(16):2020–2035.
54. Wood FO, Leonowicz NA, Vanhecke TE, Dixon SR, Grines CL. Mortality in patients with ST-segment elevation myocardial infarction who do not undergo reperfusion. *Am J Cardiol.* 2012;110(4):509–514.
55. Mixon TA, Suhr E, Caldwell G, et al. Retrospective description and analysis of consecutive catheterization laboratory ST-segment elevation myocardial infarction activations with proposal, rationale, and use of a new classification scheme. *Circ Cardiovasc Qual Outcomes.* 2012;5(1):62–69.
56. Chang AM, Shofer FS, Tabas JA, et al. Lack of association between left bundle-branch block and acute myocardial infarction in symptomatic ED patients. *Am J Emerg Med.* 2009;27(8):916–921.

57. Jain S, Ting HT, Bell M, et al. Utility of left bundle branch block as a diagnostic criterion for acute myocardial infarction. *Am J Cardiol.* 2011;107(8):1111–1116.
58. Smith SW, Dodd KW, Henry TD, Dvorak DM, Pearce LA. Diagnosis of ST-elevation myocardial infarction in the presence of left bundle branch block with the ST-elevation to S-wave ratio in a modified Sgarbossa rule. *Ann Emerg Med.* 2012;60(6):766–776.
59. Cai Q, Mehta N, Sgarbossa EB, et al. The left bundle-branch block puzzle in the 2013 ST-elevation myocardial infarction guideline: From falsely declaring emergency to denying reperfusion in a high-risk population. Are the Sgarbossa Criteria ready for prime time? *Am Heart J.* 2013;166(3):409–413.
60. Antman EM. Time is muscle: translation into practice. *J Am Coll Cardiol.* 2008;52(15):1216–1221.
61. Huber K, Goldstein P, Danchin N, et al. Enhancing the efficacy of delivering reperfusion therapy: a European and North American experience with ST-segment elevation myocardial infarction networks. *Am Heart J.* 2013;165(2):123–132.
62. Jacobs AK, Antman EM, Faxon DP, Gregory T, Solis P. Development of systems of care for ST-elevation myocardial infarction patients: Executive summary. *Circulation.* 2007;116(2):217–230.
63. Widimsky P, Fajadet J, Danchin N, Wijns W. "Stent 4 Life" targeting PCI at all who will benefit the most. A joint project between EAPCI, Euro-PCR, EUCOMED and the ESC Working Group on Acute Cardiac Care. *EuroIntervention.* 2009;4(5):555–557.
64. Nielsen PH, Terkelsen CJ, Nielsen TT, et al. System delay and timing of intervention in acute myocardial infarction (from the Danish Acute Myocardial Infarction-2 [DANAMI-2] trial). *Am J Cardiol.* 2011;108(6):776–781.
65. Le May MR, So DY, Dionne R, et al. A citywide protocol for primary PCI in ST-segment elevation myocardial infarction. *N Engl J Med.* 2008;358(3):231–240.
66. Nallamothu BK, Krumholz HM, Ko DT, et al. Development of systems of care for ST-elevation myocardial infarction patients: gaps, barriers, and implications. *Circulation.* 2007;116(2):e68–e72.
67. Fosbol EL, Granger CB, Jollis JG, et al. The impact of a statewide pre-hospital STEMI strategy to bypass hospitals without percutaneous coronary intervention capability on treatment times. *Circulation.* 2013;127(5):604–612.
68. Le May MR, Wells GA, So DY, et al. Reduction in mortality as a result of direct transport from the field to a receiving center for primary percutaneous coronary intervention. *J Am Coll Cardiol.* 2012;60(14):1223–1230.
69. Bagai A, Jollis JG, Dauerman HL, et al. Emergency department bypass for ST-segment elevation myocardial infarction patients

identified with a pre-hospital electrocardiogram: a report from the American Heart Association Mission: Lifeline Program. *Circulation.* 2013; 128(4):352-9.

70. Henry TD, Sharkey SW, Burke MN, et al. A regional system to provide timely access to percutaneous coronary intervention for ST-elevation myocardial infarction. *Circulation.* 2007;116(7):721–728.
71. Field JM, Hazinski MF, Sayre MR, et al. Part 1: Executive summary: 2010 American Heart Association Guidelines for Cardiopulmonary Resuscitation and Emergency Cardiovascular Care. *Circulation.* 2010;122(18 suppl. 3):S640–S656.
72. Dumas F, Cariou A, Manzo-Silberman S, et al. Immediate percutaneous coronary intervention is associated with better survival after out-of-hospital cardiac arrest: Insights from the PROCAT (Parisian Region Out of hospital Cardiac ArresT) Registry. *Circ Cardiovasc Interv.* 2010;3(3):200–207.
73. Kern KB. Optimal treatment of patients surviving out-of-hospital cardiac arrest. *JACC Cardiovasc Interv.* 2012;5(6):597–605.
74. Hosmane VR, Mustafa NG, Reddy VK, et al. Survival and neurologic recovery in patients with ST-segment elevation myocardial infarction resuscitated from cardiac arrest. *J Am Coll Cardiol.* 2009;53(5):409–415.
75. Gorjup V, Radsel P, Kocjancic ST, Erzen D, Noc M. Acute ST-elevation myocardial infarction after successful cardiopulmonary resuscitation. *Resuscitation.* 2007;72(3):379–385.
76. Nichol G, Aufderheide TP, Eigel B, et al. Regional systems of care for out-of-hospital cardiac arrest: A policy statement from the American Heart Association. *Circulation.* 2010;121(5):709–729.
77. Nolan JP, Soar J. Post resuscitation care–time for a care bundle? *Resuscitation.* 2008;76(2):161–162.
78. Keeley EC, Boura JA, Grines CL. Primary angioplasty versus intravenous thrombolytic therapy for acute myocardial infarction: a quantitative review of 23 randomised trials. *Lancet.* 2003;361(9351):13–20.
79. Armstrong PW, Boden WE. Reperfusion paradox in ST-segment elevation myocardial infarction. *Ann Intern Med.* 2011;155(6):389–391.
80. Bjorklund E, Stenestrand U, Lindback J, et al. Pre-hospital thrombolysis delivered by paramedics is associated with reduced time delay and mortality in ambulance-transported real-life patients with ST-elevation myocardial infarction. *Eur Heart J.* 2006;27(10):1146–1152.
81. Morrison LJ, Verbeek PR, McDonald AC, Sawadsky BV, Cook DJ. Mortality and prehospital thrombolysis for acute myocardial infarction: A meta-analysis. *JAMA.* 2000;283(20):2686–2692.
82. Huynh T, Birkhead J, Huber K, et al. The pre-hospital fibrinolysis experience in Europe and North America and implications for wider dissemination. *JACC Cardiovasc Interv.* 2011;4(8):877–883.

83. Welsh RC, Chang W, Goldstein P, et al. Time to treatment and the impact of a physician on prehospital management of acute ST elevation myocardial infarction: insights from the ASSENT-3 PLUS trial. *Heart.* 2005;91(11):1400–1406.
84. Welsh RC, Travers A, Senaratne M, Williams R, Armstrong PW. Feasibility and applicability of paramedic-based prehospital fibrinolysis in a large North American Center. *Am Heart J.* 2006;152(6):1007–1014.
85. Henry TD, Gersh BJ. Is there a role for pre-hospital fibrinolysis in North America? *JACC Cardiovasc Interv.* 2011;4(8):884–886.
86. Tubaro M, Danchin N, Goldstein P, et al. Pre-hospital treatment of STEMI patients. A scientific statement of the Working Group Acute Cardiac Care of the European Society of Cardiology. *Acute Card Care.* 2011;13(2):56–67.
87. Armstrong PW. A comparison of pharmacologic therapy with/without timely coronary intervention vs. primary percutaneous intervention early after ST-elevation myocardial infarction: the WEST (Which Early ST-elevation myocardial infarction Therapy) study. *Eur Heart J.* 2006;27(13):1530–1538.
88. Westerhout CM, Bonnefoy E, Welsh RC, et al. The influence of time from symptom onset and reperfusion strategy on 1-year survival in ST-elevation myocardial infarction: a pooled analysis of an early fibrinolytic strategy versus primary percutaneous coronary intervention from CAPTIM and WEST. *Am Heart J.* 2011;161(2):283–290.
89. Steg PG, Bonnefoy E, Chabaud S, et al. Impact of time to treatment on mortality after prehospital fibrinolysis or primary angioplasty: data from the CAPTIM randomized clinical trial. *Circulation.* 2003;108(23):2851–2856.
90. Bonnefoy E, Steg PG, Boutitie F, et al. Comparison of primary angioplasty and pre-hospital fibrinolysis in acute myocardial infarction (CAPTIM) trial: a 5-year follow-up. *Eur Heart J.* 2009;30(13):1598–1606.
91. Armstrong PW, Gershlick AH, Goldstein P, et al. Fibrinolysis or primary PCI in ST-segment elevation myocardial infarction. *N Engl J Med.* 2013;368(15):1379–1387.

CHAPTER 2

The Time Dilemma and Decision Making for Prehospital Fibrinolysis, Hospital Fibrinolysis, and/or Transfer to a Percutaneous Coronary Intervention Center

Freij Gobal, MD, Abdul Hakeem, MD, Zubair Ahmed, MD, and Barry F. Uretsky, MD

INTRODUCTION

Of all the factors associated with reducing ST-segment elevation myocardial infarction (STEMI) mortality, none is more important than early reperfusion of the infarct-related artery. Mechanical recanalization by primary percutaneous coronary intervention (PPCI) is the preferred approach, with convincing data that it is superior to fibrinolysis under most circumstances. As such, it is considered the treatment of choice with a class I indication by both American and European guidelines when treatment can be performed with a delay of less than 120 minutes.[1-4] This chapter will review the current approaches to treatment relative to the delay to treatment.

Prehospital Management of Acute STEMI: Practical Approaches and International Strategies for Early Intervention © 2015 Joseph S. Alpert, Lynne T. Braun, Barbara J. Fletcher, Gerald Fletcher, Editors-in-Chief, Cardiotext Publishing, ISBN: 978-1-935395-66-9

"TIME IS MUSCLE" AND THE "GOLDEN HOUR" FOR REPERFUSION

The "Time Course" of Necrosis

Over 50 years ago, pioneering work by Jennings et al. demonstrated the temporal histopathological changes associated with occlusion of an epicardial coronary artery in a dog model.[5,6] Reimer et al. later demonstrated the "wavefront phenomenon," the pattern of irreversible myocardial injury spreading from the subendocardium to the epicardium as a function of duration of epicardial vessel occlusion.[7] After 40 minutes of circumflex artery occlusion, 38% of the at-risk myocardium had necrosis versus 57% at 3 hours, 71% at 6 hours, and 85% of the myocardium had necrosis at 24 hours (Figure 2.1A). Salvage of 55% of the myocardium was accomplished on reperfusion at 40 minutes of occlusion versus 33% at 3 hours and 16% at 6 hours (Figure 2.1B). This model produced the concept of "at risk" myocardium and myocardial "salvage" and paved the way for employing pharmacological and mechanical interventions to reestablish reperfusion in the human infarct-related artery.[7] Over the past 3 decades, numerous clinical trials have demonstrated that the key determinant of myocardial salvage and subsequent short- and long-term outcomes is "time to reperfusion" after vessel occlusion.

Time to Fibrinolysis: "The Golden Hour"

The importance of time to pharmacological recanalization with fibrinolytic therapy has been established in multiple randomized controlled trials (RCTs). The Fibrinolytic Therapy Trialists' (FTT) Collaborative Group pooled data from 9 RCTs with 58,600 patients (10.5% mortality at 35 days).[8] Mortality reduction was greatest in patients presenting within one hour of symptom onset: the absolute benefit was 35 ± 11 additional

A

B

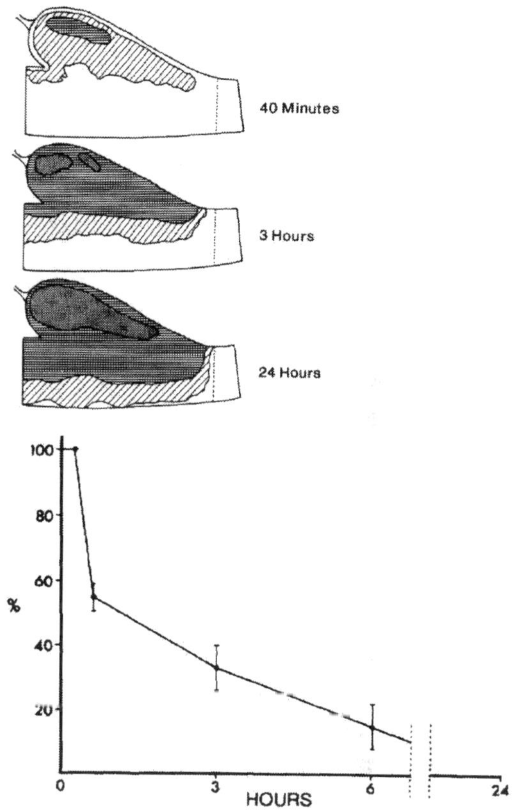

Figure 2.1

A. Progression of the ischemic wavefront of cell death from subendocardium to epicardium as a function of time. **B.** Proportion of ischemic muscle that is viable and probably salvageable as a function of time after coronary occlusion. **C** and **D.** Within the "golden hour" for reperfusion (symptom duration <2 hours, ideally <1 hour), the slope of the relation between ischemic time and outcome is extremely steep. Systematic overview of randomized, placebo-controlled trials of fibrinolysis revealed that maximum benefit was achieved when treatment was given within 60 minutes of symptom onset, which led to the concept of the "golden hour"; thereafter, benefit declined exponentially and largely flattened after 6 hours, which parallels the salvage index defined by Jennings and Reimer. (Reprinted with permission (1A and 1B)[6] and (1C and 1D).[8]

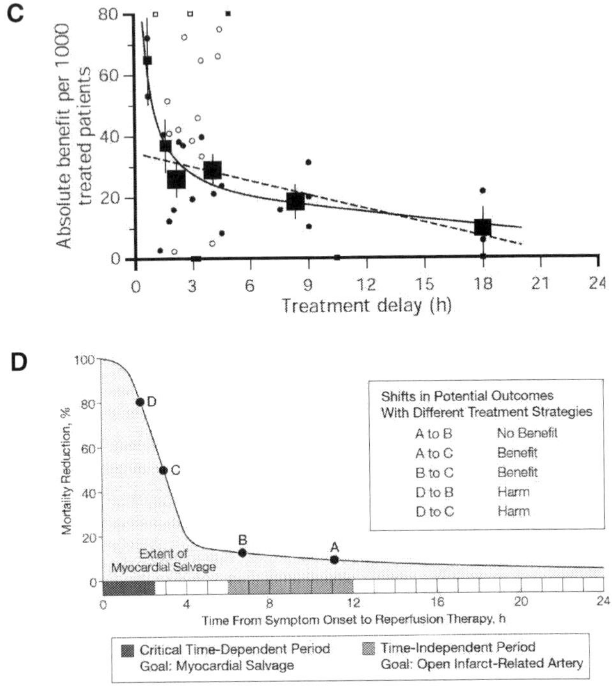

Figure 2.1

(*Continued*)

patients alive per 1000 treated. The benefits were 25 ± 5 and 19 ± 5 additional lives saved per 1000 patients for total ischemic times of 1 to 3 and 3 to 6 hours, respectively. In a separate analysis, the mortality reduction was highest in patients treated within one hour (48%), and significantly higher in patients treated within 2 hours than in those treated later (44% vs. 20%).[9] A large mortality reduction was also detected in patients treated within one hour of symptom onset (65 per 1000 treated).[9] These results have led to the concept of the "golden hour," that is, the first hour after symptom onset, during which maximal clinical benefit for fibrinolysis is achieved with the therapeutic effect declining exponentially thereafter, being essentially flat after 6 hours (Figure 2.1C and D). Reperfusion with fibrinolysis within this golden hour can lead in some cases to complete "abortion" of myocardial infarction (MI), i.e., avoidance of myocardial necrosis, as demonstrated in an analysis from the Assessment of the Safety and Efficacy of a New Thrombolytic agent (ASSENT-3) trial.[10] Seven hundred and twenty seven (13.3%) of 5470 patients had an aborted MI, i.e., achieved complete resolution (≥ 70%) of their initial ST-elevation with minimal or no myocardial enzyme elevation indicative of necrosis.[10] Fibrinolysis within one hour of symptom onset led to MI abortion in 25% of patients with an exponential decrement in benefit thereafter with only 10% aborted MIs in the > 3 hours group.

Time to PPCI

Time to revascularization is equally important for achieving the maximal clinical benefit from PPCI. In a Global Use of Strategies to Open Occluded Arteries in Acute Coronary Syndromes (GUSTO) IIb substudy, 30 day mortality rate was lowest in patients undergoing PPCI within 60 minutes from symptom onset to emergency room arrival, whereas the highest mortality rate occurred in patients undergoing PPCI > 90 minutes (1.0% vs. 6.4%).[11] Similar compelling "real-world" evidence was provided from the National Registry of Acute MI (NRMI) analysis of more than 27,000 patients with the lowest mortality rate observed in patients undergoing PPCI within 60 minutes from presentation and higher mortality rates observed in patients undergoing PPCI beyond 120 minutes (multivariate-adjusted odds of mortality were approximately 40% to 60% higher for > 2 hours).[12] In another NRMI-3 analysis, longer door-to-device (DTD) times were associated with increased in-hospital mortality (mortality rate of 3.0%, 4.2%, 5.7%, and 7.4% for DTD times of ≤ 90 minutes, 91 to 120 minutes,

121 to 150 minutes, and > 150 minutes, respectively [P for trend < 0.01]).[12] De Luca demonstrated a 7.5% increase in one-year mortality for every 30-minute increase in time from symptom onset to PPCI.[13] Given the time dependency of survival in STEMI patients undergoing PPCI, the American College of Cardiology (ACC) and American Heart Association (AHA) guidelines for STEMI management have established a DTD of 90 minutes as the maximally acceptable time from hospital entry ("door") to first device treatment.[1]

Relative Time Dependency of PPCI Versus Fibrinolysis

While it has been well established that very early perfusion (the "golden hour") can lead to MI abortion and dramatic reduction in total mortality, the time dependency for efficacy of various reperfusion therapies may be quite different (Figure 2.2).[14] Fibrinolysis is more sensitive to time delay versus PPCI, which in turn is primarily related to thrombus organization. With increasing time after clot development, the amount of cross-linked fibrin increases, thereby promoting resistance to fibrinolysis. In a meta-analysis of 10 RCTs, the median time from randomization to PPCI was 69 versus 22 minutes for fibrinolysis.[10] Despite shorter time to treatment in the fibrinolysis arm, PPCI patients had a lower rate of major adverse events compared to fibrinolysis patients, both at 30 days and at 6 months (Figure 2.3A and B). Furthermore, there was a significant increase in the major adverse event rate in fibrinolysis patients with increasing time to presentation, whereas in PPCI patients, the major adverse events rate remained relatively stable. The Stent versus Thrombolysis for Occluded coronary arteries in Patients with Acute MI (STOP AMI) trial similarly concluded that the extent of salvage is less dependent on the passage of time with PPCI than fibrinolysis.[15]

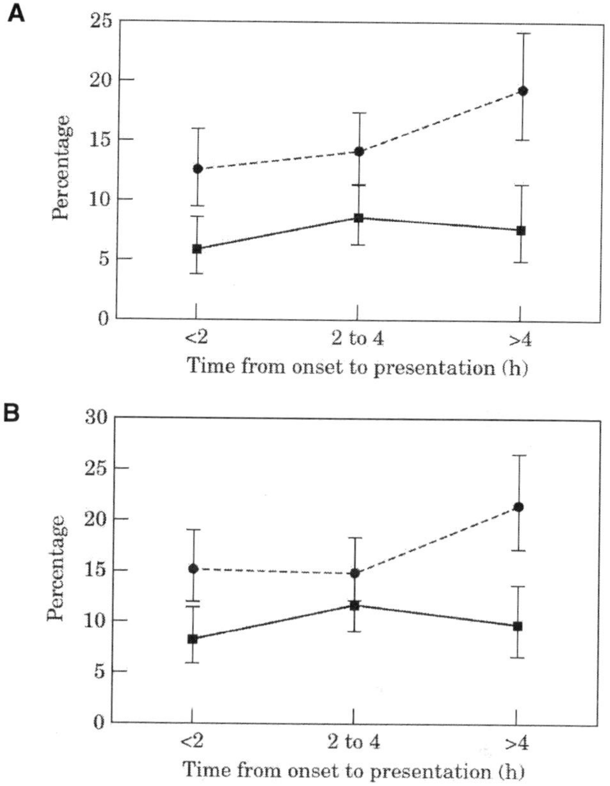

Figure 2.2

Time dependency of PPCI versus fibrinolysis. Rate of death and non-fatal reinfarction at 30 days **(A)** and 6 months **(B)** (with 95% confidence intervals) in patients presenting early (< 2 h), intermediate (2–4 h) and late (> 4 h). Dotted line and circles, fibrinolysis; Straight line and boxes, PPCI (Reprinted with permission).[14]

PPCI-Related Time Delay

An estimated 40% of STEMI patients in the United States present to non-PPCI capable hospitals.[16] Given the benefit of PPCI over fibrinolytic therapy, RCTs have validated a transfer strategy for PPCI as superior to on-site fibrinolytic therapy.

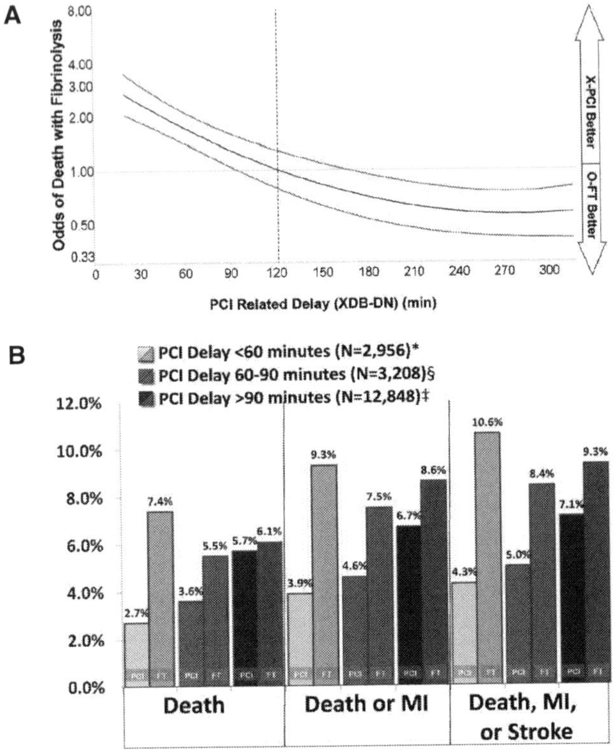

Figure 2.3

A. Relationship between PPCI-related delay (minutes) and in-hospital mortality. Dotted lines represent 95% confidence intervals. XDB-DN indicates transfer delay (transfer door-to-balloon minus DTN time).
B. Clinical outcomes among matched patients stratified by PCI-related delay. FT, fibrinolytic therapy; MI, myocardial infarction. (Reprinted with permission).[19]

In a meta-analysis of 11 trials comprising 5741 patients comparing a transfer strategy to on-site fibrinolysis, a transfer strategy was associated with a significant reduction in 30-day mortality, reinfarction, and stroke independent of time delay to PPCI.[17] However, controversy persists as to the length of a PPCI-related delay that is safe and more effective than fibrinolysis alone.[9,16–19] One regression meta-analysis of RCTs by Nallamothu et al. suggested that PPCI-related mortality benefit may be lost when a PPCI-related time delay [DTD minus door-to-needle (DTN) time] is >60 minutes compared with immediate administration of a fibrin-specific lytic agent,[9] but other studies have not confirmed this time threshold; some even suggest that up to 3 hours may not negate the net clinical benefit of PPCI over fibrinolysis.[16–19]

A NRMI database study, using a propensity-score matched analysis of over 19,000 patients who underwent on-site fibrinolysis versus transfer for PPCI,[19] showed that the magnitude of the PPCI mortality benefit exponentially decreased as time delay to PPCI increased (number needed to treat, 23 for PPCI-related delay <60 minutes; 44 for PPCI-related delay 60–90 minutes; 250 for PPCI-related delay >90 minutes). When delay exceeded 120 minutes, the PPCI mortality advantage was lost, and when delay exceeded 160 minutes, the benefit on the combination of death, MI, and stroke was lost. The absolute benefit of a PPCI transfer strategy was greater among those presenting between 2 and 6 hours from symptom onset compared with <2 hours, suggesting an enhanced benefit of transfer strategy for PPCI over fibrinolysis with longer prehospital delay (Figure 2.3A).[19] Additionally, at no point was survival with transfer strategy inferior to fibrinolysis (Figure 2.3B). The 2013 ACCF/AHA STEMI guidelines update have extended the acceptable DTD time to 120 minutes for patients presenting to non-PPCI-capable hospitals in agreement with the European guidelines.[1,2]

THERAPEUTIC OPTIONS WITH ANTICIPATED DELAY TO PPCI OF >90 TO 120 MINUTES

A primary goal in improving STEMI care in healthcare systems of various countries is to create methods to minimize time between onset of symptoms and PPCI. However, early PPCI may not always be possible. This section reviews options when the expected DTD time is >90 to 120 minutes.

Fibrinolysis with "Rescue PCI" as Needed

Fibrinolysis was firmly established in 1988 when the Second International Study of Infarct Survival (ISIS-2) trial showed a mortality relative risk reduction of 25% in streptokinase versus placebo patients who were treated <24 hours after onset of symptoms. The therapeutic benefit persisted for at least 10 years after treatment.[20,21] Subsequent studies have shown relatively higher efficacy with fibrin-specific agents such as alteplase[22] and tenecteplase (TNK).[23] Meta-analysis of 9 fibrinolytic trials showed an 18% relative reduction in short-term mortality versus placebo.[8] The 2013 ACCF/AHA STEMI guidelines update provides a class I indication for fibrinolysis if the DTD delay with PPCI is expected to be >120 minutes.[1]

There are, however, well-known limitations to fibrinolytic use in addition to absolute contraindications such as bleeding diathesis. Hemorrhagic stroke risk remains approximately 2 times higher than PPCI.[3] There is either incomplete or no reperfusion in 30% to 50% of cases.[24–26] Reocclusion after successful fibrinolysis is often symptomatic with adverse outcomes.[27–30] According to the 2004 ACC/AHA STEMI guidelines,[31] fibrinolysis may not be as effective in patients with cardiogenic shock, severe congestive heart failure (CHF), ventricular arrhythmias, previously failed fibrinolytic therapy,[32] prior MI,[33] and prior coronary artery bypass grafting (CABG).[34]

If there is evidence of failed reperfusion or reocclusion after fibrinolytic therapy, it is an ACCF/AHA guideline class IIa recommendation to urgently transfer STEMI patients to a PCI-capable hospital for "rescue PCI."[1] This recommendation is based on evidence that rescue PCI is more effective than conservative therapy or repeat fibrinolysis. In the Middlesbrough Early Vascularization to Limit Infarction trial, patients who failed fibrinolysis, as demonstrated by < 50% ECG ST-segment resolution at 60 minutes, were randomized to either rescue PCI or conservative treatment.[35] Although there was no mortality difference at 30 days, event-free survival was improved primarily due to a reduction in subsequent revascularization. However, stroke rate (4.6% vs. 0.6%) and need for transfusion (11.1% vs. 1.3%) were higher with rescue PCI. At one year follow-up,[36] further revascularization was significantly lower in the rescue PCI group with no mortality difference. The Rescue Angioplasty versus Conservative Treatment or Repeat Thrombolysis (REACT) trial randomized 427 patients with failed reperfusion (defined as < 50% ST-segment resolution within 90 minutes after fibrinolysis) to repeat fibrinolysis, conservative treatment, or rescue PCI.[37] Rescue PCI had a higher event-free survival (84.6%) compared with repeated thrombolysis or conservative treatment (68.7% and 70.1%, respectively). In a meta-analysis by Wijeysundera,[38] rescue PCI was associated with improved outcomes for heart failure, reinfarction, and the composite end point of all-cause mortality, heart failure, or reinfarction. However, there was a small but statistically significant increase (3%) in absolute stroke risk.

In summary, rescue PCI is associated with improved clinical outcomes for STEMI patients if used subsequent for failed fibrinolysis, but these benefits must be interpreted in the context of potential risks.

The Undelivered Promise of "Facilitated" PCI (Immediate Fibrinolytic Therapy Followed by PPCI)

A theoretically ideal alternative to minimize time to reperfuse the "culprit" occlusion is the strategy of using either fibrinolytic therapy (half or full dose) or half-dose fibrinolytic with a glycoprotein (GP) IIb/IIIa inhibitor followed by PPCI. This strategy, known as "facilitated" PCI, has been tested against fibrinolysis alone[39–45] and PPCI.[46–53] In both scenarios, this approach, despite theoretical appeal, was relatively ineffective. Compared with fibrinolytics alone, it was ineffective except for a decrease in revascularization in some studies.[3,20,46–48] However, bleeding risk was clearly worse (Tables 2.1–2.3).

In a meta-analysis of 17 trials, there was no advantage for facilitated versus PPCI.[54] Conversely, studies using regimens that included fibrinolytic drugs alone without a GP IIb/IIIa inhibitor suggested an increased risk of death, nonfatal reinfarction, urgent target vessel revascularization, bleeding, and stroke, influenced to a great extent by the ASSENT-4 study.[54] The Facilitated Intervention with Enhanced Reperfusion Speed to Stop Events (FINESSE) trial randomized 2452 patients in a 1:1:1 ratio to reduced-dose reteplase plus abciximab (combination-facilitated PCI), abciximab alone (abciximab-facilitated PCI), or placebo (PPCI).[55] The composite of death from all causes, ventricular fibrillation occurring >48 hours after randomization, cardiogenic shock, and heart failure during the first 90 days after randomization was essentially the same in all groups, even though significantly more patients in the combination facilitated-PCI group had >70% ST-segment resolution at 60 to 90 minutes and significantly greater percentage of angiographic Thrombolysis In Myocardial Infarction (TIMI) 3 flow pre-PPCI.

According to the 2007 ACC/AHA focus STEMI update, facilitated PCI using regimens other than full-dose fibrinolytic therapy holds a IIb recommendation if the patient is at high risk, has alow bleeding risk, and PPCI is not immediately available.[56] This approach, however, is considered class III (not helpful or may be harmful) using full-dose fibrinolytic therapy followed by PPCI.[56]

Table 2.1
Thrombolytics compared to facilitated PCI

Trial	(Citation)	Year	N		Death			Reinfarction			Revascularization			Bleeding		
			T	F	T	F	*P*	T	F	*P*	T	F	*P*	T	F	*P*
Vermeer	(38)	1999	75	74	6.7%	8.1%	NS	9.3%	5.4%	NS	30.7%	23.0%	NS	11%	21%	NR
PRAGUE	(39)	2000	99	100	14%	12%	NS	10%	7%	NS	14.1%	7%	NS	0%	7.2%	<0.001
GUSTO-4 SPEED	(40)	2000	162	323	3.7%	3.4%	1.00	4.9%	1.2%	0.03	9.3%	1.6%	0.001	8.6%	6.5%	0.46
TIMI 10B – TIMI 14	(41)	2001	738	1,200	3%	3%	NR	3%	3%	NR		NR			NR	
SIAM III	(42)	2003	81	82	9.9%	4.9%	0.17	2.5%	2.4%	0.68	2.5%	2.4%	0.68	7.4%	9.8%	0.40
GRACIA-1	(43)	2004	252	248	2%	2%	0.84	2%	1%	0.98	12%	2%	0.0001	1.6%	1.6%	NS
CAPITAL AMI	(44)	2005	84	86	3.6%	2.3%	0.68	13.3%	4.7%	0.06	50.6%	13.9%	0.001	13.1%	23.3%	0.11

F, facilitated PCI; N, number of patients; NR, not reported; NS, not significant; OR, odds ratio; *P*, level of statistical significance; T, thrombolytics only; Year, year of publication.

Table 2.2
PPCI compared to full-dose lytic-facilitated PCI

			N		Death			Reinfarction			Revascularization			Bleeding		
Trial	(citation)	Year	Pr	F	Pr	F	*P*	Pr	F	*P*	Pr	F	*P*	Pr	F	*P*
Vermeer	(41)	1999	75	74	6.7%	8.1%	NS	1.3%	5.4%	NS	6%	23.0%	NS	11%	21%	N
PRAGUE	(42)	2000	101	100	7%	12%	NS	1%	7%	<0.03	6.9%	7%	NS	0%	7.2%	<0.001
Kurihara	(46)	2004	20	19	0%	0%	NS	5%	5.8%	NS	31.6%	17.6%	NS	0%	0%	NS
Möckel	(47)	2005	44	53	4.5%	20.9%	0.028	0%	2.9%	NS	2.3%	0%	NS	2.3%	11.4%	NS
ASSENT-4	(48)	2006	838	829	5%	7%	0.14	4%	6%	0.027	3%	7%	0.0041	4.4%	5.6%	0.31

F, facilitated PCI; N, number of patients; NS, not significant; Pr, primary PCI; *P*, level of statistical significance; Year, year of publication.

Table 2.3
PPCI compared to reduced-dose lytic-facilitated PCI

Trial	(Citation)	Year	N		Death			Reinfarction			Revascularization			Bleeding		
			Pr	F-r	Pr	F-r	*P*	Pr	F-r	*P*	Pr	F-r	*P*	Pr	F-r	*P*
PACT	(49)	1999	304	302	3.3%	3.6%	0.81	2.6%	3%	0.80	7.2%	7.3%	0.98	13.5%	12.9%	0.84
Dudek	(50)	2003	-	200	-	3.5%	-	-	1%	-	-	1.5%	-	-	3%	-
BRAVE	(51)	2004	128	125	1.6%	1.6%	NR	0%	0.8%	NR	NR	NR	NR	1.6%	5.6%	0.16
Maioli	(52)	2005	99	113	6.1%	6.3%	0.19	NR	NR	NR	1%	0%	0.56	3%	6.2%	0.22
ADVANCE MI	(53)	2005	74	74	0%	7%	0.03	3%	1%	0.33	NR	NR	NR	7%	23%	0.05

F-r, reduced-dose facilitated PCI; N, number of patients; NR, not reported; Pr, primary PCI; *P*, level of statistical significance; Year, year of publication.

"Pharmacoinvasive" Approach: Is it an Advance?

The pharmacoinvasive (PI) approach is defined as routine administration of a pharmacologic agent (fibrinolytic therapy with or without a GP IIb/IIIa inhibitor) prior to planned PCI. The planned PCI in this strategy is usually performed 3 to 24 hours after pharmacological treatment, unlike facilitated PCI, in which PCI is performed as early as possible after fibrinolytic therapy. It carries a class IIa recommendation in both American and European guidelines[1,2] based on 3 major RCTs demonstrating that, when compared to pharmacological therapy alone and performing PCI only as "rescue" for failed thrombolysis, routine planned PCI after pharmacotherapy was effective in improving short- and long-term outcomes (Table 2.4).[57–59] Wijeysundera[60] reviewed 5 PI trials which included 1235 patients followed for 30 days to one year. Patients randomized to routine invasive strategy, with weighted average time from fibrinolytic to PCI of 8.4 hours, had significant reductions in mortality and reinfarction compared with ischemia-guided management. Importantly, there were no significant differences in the risk of stroke or major bleeding. Most recently, the STREAM trial randomized 1892 patients with symptoms of < 3 hours to early (prehospital or emergency room) fibrinolysis (with TNK) followed by early (6–24 hours) angiography and intervention or rescue angioplasty versus PPCI where delay to intervention was expected to be > 60 minutes.[81] The primary composite end point of death, cardiogenic shock, heart failure, or reintervention by 30 days was similar, emphasizing the value of very early fibrinolytic therapy, particularly when PPCI will be relatively delayed (in this study, median delay for PPCI was 86 minutes).

Table 2.4
Pharmacoinvasive therapy compared with fibrinolysis + PCI for rescue only

Trial	(Citation)	Year	Treatment Group	Control Group	N	Primary End-Point	*P*
CARESS-in-AMI	(57)	2008	Half-dose reteplase and abciximab + PCI within 6 hours	Half-dose reteplase and abciximab only	598	Composite of death, re-MI, or refractory ischemia at 30 days: 4% versus 11%	0.004
TRANSFER-AMI	(58)	2009	Tenecteplase + PCI within 6 hours	Tenecteplase only	1059	Composite of death, re-MI, recurrent ischemia, CHF, or cardiogenic shock at 20 days: 11% versus 17%	0.004
NORDISTEMI	(59)	2010	Tenecteplase + PCI within 6 hours	Tenecteplase only	266	Composite of death, re-MI, stroke or new ischemia at 12 months: 21% versus 27%	0.19

N, number of patients; *P*, level of statistical significance; Year, year of publication.

Can the Time "Window" for PPCI Be Opened Wider?

It is uncertain whether PPCI is the best therapy when a time delay of greater than 90 to 120 minutes is expected in patients who present beyond the first few hours of symptom onset, as RCTs have not evaluated PPCI after that time delay.

The Register of Information and Knowledge About Swedish Heart Intensive Care Admissions (RIKS-HIA) investigators reviewed the outcomes of 26,205 patients treated with reperfusion therapy.[61] The median symptom-to-needle and symptom-to-device times were 120 minutes for patients receiving prehospital fibrinolysis, 167 minutes for in-hospital fibrinolysis, and 210 minutes for PPCI. Despite a longer delay, PPCI was associated with significantly lower early and late mortality than either prehospital or in-hospital fibrinolysis. PPCI also resulted in significantly lower rates of both early and late reinfarction and reduced length of stay. The study concluded that PPCI mortality benefits are >20% in the early hours after symptom onset and increase to 30% to 35% in the later hours, and that not until a delay of 6 to 7 hours does the mortality of PPCI become comparable with that of fibrinolysis administered within the first hours. Pinto examined outcomes from 192,509 NRMI patients at 645 hospitals treated with either PPCI or fibrinolysis. Mortality after PPCI remained lower until a PPCI-related delay of 114 minutes was reached.[62]

ADJUNCTIVE PREHOSPITAL PHARMACOTHERAPY

Aspirin

A platelet-rich thrombus lies at the epicenter of an acutely occluded epicardial vessel. Besides obstructing flow, it contributes toward microvascular dysfunction and vascular inflammation. Activated platelets release thromboxane A2 (TXA2), which induces platelet aggregation through a G-protein-coupled TXA2 receptor. Aspirin is effective in preventing much of the platelet's thrombogenic effect by irreversibly acetylating and inhibiting COX-1, a critical enzyme in the biosynthesis of TXA2.

Administration of oral or sublingual aspirin prehospitalization as early as possible, either by the patient or emergency personnel, is the standard of care (class I), codified in both the ACCF/AHA and ESC guidelines with a strong (Level A) evidence base.[1,2] For patients unable to take oral aspirin, intravenous aspirin dose is recommended by ESC 2013 guidelines. The ISIS-2 study, the largest aspirin trial in STEMI patients, provided very strong evidence that aspirin significantly reduces mortality (relative risk reduction 23% vs. placebo).[20] The mortality benefit was additive to the 25% relative risk reduction from streptokinase such that combined use reduced mortality (compared with either agent alone) by 42%.

A larger dose of aspirin (162–325 mg) should be given initially as lower doses (40–80 mg) may require several days to achieve full antiplatelet effects. For earliest onset of antiplatelet effects, aspirin should be chewed to allow for buccal absorption.

Thienopyridines

Despite COX-1 inhibition by aspirin, platelet activation may still occur through TXA2-independent pathways. Thienopyridine inhibition of the platelet P2Y12 ADP surface receptor is another mechanism to decrease platelet effectiveness in promoting thrombosis. The use of dual antiplatelet therapy (DAPT, aspirin plus a thienopyridine) is well established as providing the best outcomes in the setting of routine stenting.[63] Based on RCTs, 3 thienopyridines, clopidogrel, prasugrel, and ticagrelor, have a class I indication.[64–67] These agents differ in their onset of action and degree of platelet inhibition. Guidelines recommend that if PPCI is considered, a thienopyridine be given "as early as possible";[1,2] that is, it may be administered during hospital transit or transfer. There is a paucity of RCT data comparing DAPT therapy prehospitalization versus on-arrival. Because of the time delay of onset of drug action, it has been common practice in Europe to administer the drug preangiography to achieve better efficacy. Some concerns have been raised about this strategy insofar as a small percentage of patients undergoing angiography may require, in addition to PPCI, emergency or very urgent surgery and that surgery with DAPT on board portends an increased bleeding risk.

GP IIb/IIIa Inhibitor

The GP IIb/IIIa inhibitors are powerful inhibitors of platelet aggregation by blocking the primary receptor for platelet-to-platelet aggregation, the platelet IIb/IIIa surface receptor. There are some data supporting prehospital GP IIb/IIIa inhibitor administration but no large RCTs. A meta-analysis of 11 randomized trials of 27,115 patients suggested abciximab may reduce reinfarction and mortality rates at 30 days.[68] The On-TIME 2 study randomized 1398 patients to the prehospital use of tirofiban versus placebo with DAPT for all and demonstrated that tirofiban decreased the extent of residual ST-segment deviation and improved ST-segment resolution 1 hour after PCI as well as improved clinical outcome at 30 days and one year compared with no tirofiban treatment, although the study was not powered for clinical events.[69] At one year, there was a trend towards mortality benefit (3.7% tirofiban vs. 5.8% no tirofiban; odds ratio (OR): 0.63; 95% CI: 0.38 to 1.06, $P = 0.08$). The Abciximab before Direct Angioplasty and Stenting in MI Regarding Acute and Long-Term (ADMIRAL) trial randomized 300 patients either to very early abciximab plus stenting or placebo plus stenting.[70] Many patients received abciximab prehospitalization in a "mobile ICU," but neither the percentage treated prehospitalization nor outcomes based on prehospital use versus in-hospital administration are provided in the publication. At 30 days, the primary composite end point of death, recurrent MI, or urgent target vessel revascularization was lower with abciximab (6.0%) versus placebo (14.6%, $P = 0.01$); at 6 months, the primary end points were 7.4% and 15.9%, respectively ($P = 0.02$). More recent trials with early thienopyridine loading have shown little to no benefit with the upstream use of a GP IIb/IIIa inhibitor. In the Bavarian Reperfusion AlternatiVes Evaluation (BRAVE) 3 trial, 800 patients, all receiving DAPT, did not demonstrate smaller infarct size or fewer ischemic end points with abciximab compared with placebo.[71] Further studies consistently demonstrate a higher risk of bleeding with GP IIb/IIIa inhibitors. The data from the BRAVE-3 and the FINESSE trial previously described, suggest limited benefit of preprocedure/prehospitalization initiation of a GP IIb/IIIa inhibitor, particularly with early DAPT institution. Both the 2013 ACCF/AHA and 2012 ESC STEMI guidelines provide a IIA indication for the use of GP IIb/IIIa inhibitor during PPCI but only a IIB indication for early administration because of the uncertain risk: benefit ratio in this setting.

Fibrinolysis in the Prehospital Setting

Information regarding emergency medical personnel administration of prehospital fibrinolytic is limited. One study has suggested some benefit for prehospital fibrinolysis versus the longer expected delay with PPCI within the 90 to 120 minutes window. The CAPTIM study was designed to compare prehospital fibrinolysis, with transfer for rescue angioplasty if needed, versus PPCI.[72] A trend toward lower mortality at 30 days was observed in the prehospital fibrinolysis group, especially in patients managed within the first 2 hours, which was maintained at 5-year follow-up.[73] These data suggest that very early fibrinolytic therapy may perform as well as PPCI, although the data are limited to a single, prematurely terminated trial. The Which Early ST-elevation MI Therapy (WEST) trial demonstrated that prehospital fibrinolysis with TNK may be comparable to TNK plus <24 hours invasive study with PCI if the vessel was still closed in terms of a combined endpoint at 30 days.[74] However, it was inferior to PPCI for 30-day death plus MI (13.0% vs. 4.0% respectively, $P = 0.02$). Very early TNK administration (20% prehospitalization) was ineffective in improving outcomes compared with PPCI in the ASSENT-4 PCI trial.[47] The Swedish RIKS-HIA Registry, as noted above, suggested that PPCI was superior to prehospital as well as in-hospital fibrinolysis in regards to 30 day and one-year mortality.[61]

Routine fibrinolytic use on first medical contact (FMC) has many challenges, including the costs of emergency medical service (EMS) personnel training, installation of computer-assisted ECG machines, and wireless transmission. Prehospital lytic therapy may be reasonable if there is a long transit time, a short period between symptom onset and treatment, and certainty about the diagnosis, which usually means formal ECG reading by a trained individual and ascertainment that MI "masqueraders" such as dissecting aneurysm are not the symptom cause. The latter suggests the importance of physician evaluation in this process. In the absence of convincing data, use of prehospital fibrinolysis should be limited and performed under a clear protocol with data collection and evaluation. The ACCF/AHA 2013 guidelines suggest the possibility that prehospital fibrinolysis may be of value but state further studies are required.[1]

Nitroglycerin

If emergency personnel determine that a STEMI is in progress with ischemic pain, and that the systemic blood pressure is normal or high, sublingual nitroglycerin with careful observation of the systemic blood pressure might be tried. Routine use of intravenous nitroglycerin during STEMI may actually increase infarct size if systemic blood pressure is excessively lowered.[75] There are no RCTs demonstrating efficacy for routine nitrate use, either prehospital or in-hospital, nor comparing intravenous, transdermal, and oral. As such, nitrates should be reserved for pain relief.

Oxygen

Oxygen is recommended at FMC including emergency transport, although in the absence of hypoxemia there are few data supporting its therapeutic value. The ACCF/AHA 2013 guidelines limit the use of supplemental oxygen on FMC for a saturation of < 90% on pulse oximetry, whereas the ESC guidelines recommend it for all patients. There has been concern that hyperoxia in patients with normal saturation may precipitate vasoconstriction of coronary arteries[76] and increase in coronary vascular resistance.[77]

Thrombin Inhibitors

Thrombin inhibitors in the STEMI and PPCI setting include unfractionated heparin (UFH), low molecular weight heparin (LMWH), and the direct thrombin inhibitor bivalirudin. UFH targets factor IIa, and to some extent, factor Xa, leading to enzymatic inactivation of thrombin. Although UFH is the primary anticoagulant used worldwide, there are no RCTs versus placebo supporting its efficacy, either prehospital or immediately after hospital entry without additional fibrinolytic therapy. Both ACCF/AHA and ESC guidelines give a class I recommendation based on expert consensus. LMWH provides the advantage of a consistent anticoagulant effect based on dose and a high anti-Xa to anti-IIa inhibitory activity.

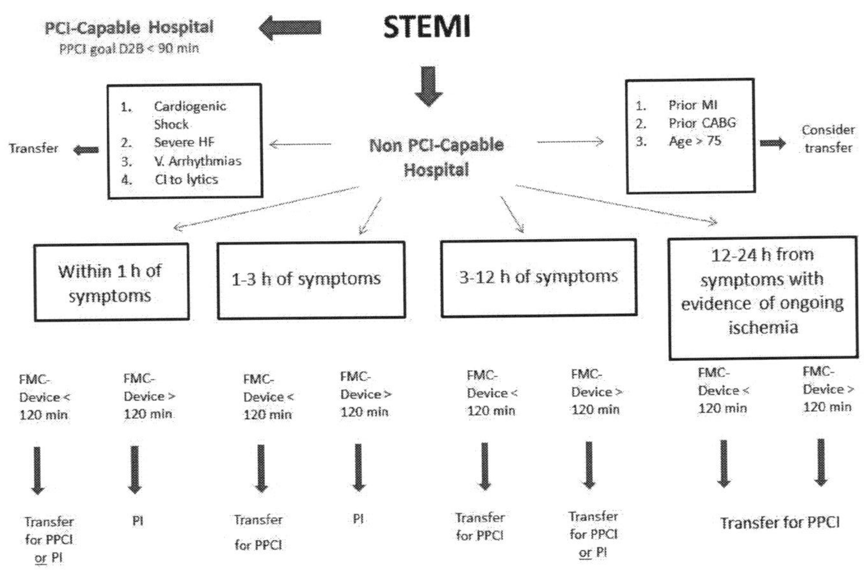

Figure 2.4

Algorithm of STEMI management in patients presenting to non-PCI capable hospitals based on expected time delay to treatment. CI, contraindication; FMC, first medical contact; PI, pharmacoinvasive therapy (for definition please refer to text); PPCI, primary percutaneous coronary intervention; STEMI, ST-elevation myocardial infarction; V, arrhythmias, ventricular arrhythmias.

Prehospital LMWH was compared to UFH as an adjunct to the fibrinolytic TNK in the ASSENT-3 Plus trial.[78] There were no significant differences in primary efficacy and safety end points. The LMWH group trended to lower in-hospital reinfarctions and refractory ischemia but increased cerebrovascular events. In the ExTRACT-TIMI 25 trial,[79] patients received fibrinolytic therapy on hospital arrival and were randomized to UFH versus LMWH. LMWH showed significant risk reduction on reinfarction and need for urgent revascularization at 30 days. The ATOLL trial randomized prehospitalized use of open-label LMWH (initially IV, followed by subcutaneous) or UFH.[80] There was a trend favoring LMWH for reduced clinical ischemic outcomes without a major difference in bleeding.

CONCLUSION

Timely reperfusion is critical in treating STEMI. However, in the "real world," there are substantial challenges to the effective implementation of this goal. The dilemma in making the best decisions in STEMI management is related, but is not limited to, time from symptom onset, anticipated time to treatment, patient risk factors, residual R waves on the ECG, and hospital volume and expertise with PPCI. Coordinated teams of interprofessional healthcare personnel need to be developed.Overall, at present, the best alternative strategy to PPCI, when treatment delay is greater than 120 minutes, is the PI approach in which fibrinolysis therapy is instituted in the emergency hospital setting, followed by transfer to a facility where PPCI is available with intervention between 3 and 24 hours thereafter. Figure 2.4 provides a detailed algorithm to guide therapy of STEMI patients, keeping in mind that institution-specific protocols reflecting current guidelines are essential.

REFERENCES

1. O'Gara PT, Kushner FG, Ascheim DD, et al. ACCF/AHA guideline for the management of ST-elevation myocardial infarction: A report of the American College of Cardiology Foundation/American Heart Association task force on practice guidelines. *J Am Coll Cardiol.* 2013;61:e78–e140.
2. Steg G, James SK, Atar D, et al. ESC guidelines for the management of acute myocardial infarction in patients presenting with ST-segment elevation. *Eur Heart J.* 2012;33:2569–2619.
3. Keeley EC, Boura JA, Grines CL. Primary angioplasty versus intravenous thrombolytic therapy for acute myocardial infarction: A quantitative review of 23 randomised trials. *Lancet.* 2003;361:13–20.
4. de Boer SP, Barnes EH, Westerhout CM, et al. High-risk patients with ST-elevation myocardial infarction derive greatest absolute benefit from primary percutaneous coronary intervention: results from the primary coronary angioplasty trialist versus thrombolysis (PCAT)-2 collaboration. *Am Heart J.* 2011;161:500–507.
5. Jenning RB, Sommers H, Smyth GA, Flack HA, Linn H. Myocardial necrosis induced by temporary occlusion of a coronary artery in the dog. *Arch Pathol.* 1960;70:68–78.
6. Jennings RB, Reimer KA. Factors involved in salvaging ischemic myocardium: effect of reperfusion of arterial blood. *Circulation.* 1983;68(pt 2):I25–I36.
7. Reimer KA, Lowe JE, Rasmussen MM, Jennings RB. The wavefront phenomenon of ischemic cell death. 1. Myocardial infarct size vs duration of coronary occlusion in dogs. *Circulation.* 1977;56:786–794.
8. Fibrinolytic Therapy Trialists' (FTT) Collaborative Group. Indications for fibrinolytic therapy in suspected acute myocardial infarction: collaborative overview of early mortality and major morbidity results from all randomized trials of more than 1000 patients. *Lancet.* 1994;343:311–322.
9. Nallamothu BK, Bates ER, Herrin J, et al. Times to treatment in transfer patients undergoing primary percutaneous coronary intervention in the United States: National Registry of Myocardial Infarction (NRMI)-3/4 Analysis. *Circulation.* 2005;111:761–767.
10. Taher T, Fu Y, Wagner GS, et al. Aborted myocardial infarction in patients with ST-segment elevation: insights from the Assessment of the Safety and Efficacy of a New Thrombolytic Regimen-3 Trial electrocardiographic sub study. *J Am Coll Cardiol.* 2004;44:38–43.
11. Berger PB, Ellis SG, Holmes DR Jr, et al. Relationship between delay in performing direct coronary angioplasty and early clinical outcome in patients with acute myocardial infarction: results from the Global Use of Strategies to Open Occluded Arteries in Acute Coronary Syndromes (GUSTO-IIb) trial. *Circulation.* 1999;100:14–20.

12. Cannon CP, Gibson CM, Lambrew CT, et al. Relationship of symptom-onset-to-balloon time and door-to-balloon time with mortality in patients undergoing angioplasty for acute myocardial infarction. *JAMA*. 2000;283:2941–2947.
13. De Luca G, Suryapranata H, Ottervanger JP, Antman EM. Time delay to treatment and mortality in primary angioplasty for acute myocardial infarction. *Circulation*. 2004;109:1223–1225.
14. Zijlstra F, Patel A, Jones M, et al. Clinical characteristics and outcome of patients with early (<2 h), intermediate (2–4 h) and late (>4 h) presentation treated by primary coronary angioplasty or thrombolytic therapy for acute myocardial infarction. *Eur Heart J*. 2002;23:550–557.
15. Schömig A, Kastrati A, Dirschinger J, et al. Coronary stenting plus platelet glycoprotein IIb/IIIa blockade compared with tissue plasminogen activator in acute myocardial infarction. Stent versus Thrombolysis for Occluded Coronary Arteries in Patients with Acute Myocardial Infarction Study Investigators. *N Engl J Med*. 2000;343:385–391.
16. Nallamothu BK, Bates ER. Percutaneous coronary intervention versus fibrinolytic therapy in acute myocardial infarction: is timing (almost) everything? *Am J Cardiol*. 2003;92:824–826.
17. De Luca G, Biondi-Zoccai G, Marino P. Transferring patients with ST-segment elevation myocardial infarction for mechanical reperfusion: a meta-regression analysis of randomized trials. *Ann Emerg Med*. 2008;52:665–676.
18. Nallamothu BK, Antman EM, Bates ER. Primary percutaneous coronary intervention versus fibrinolytic therapy in acute myocardial infarction: does the choice of fibrinolytic agent impact on the importance of time-to-treatment? *Am J Cardiol*. 2004;94:772–774.
19. Pinto DS, Frederick PD, Chakrabarti AK, et al. The benefit of transferring ST-segment–elevation myocardial infarction patients for percutaneous coronary intervention compared with administration of onsite fibrinolytic declines as delays increase. *Circulation*. 2011;124:2512–2521.
20. ISIS-2 (Second International Study of Infarct Survival) Collaborative Group. Randomised trial of intravenous streptokinase, oral aspirin, both, or neither among 17,187 cases of suspected acute myocardial infarction: ISIS-2 *Lancet*. 1988;2:349–360.
21. Baigent C, Collins R, Appleby P, et al. ISIS2: 10 year survival among patients with suspected acute myocardial infarction in randomised comparison of intravenous streptokinase, oral aspirin, both, or neither. *BMJ*. 1998;316:1337–1343.
22. GUSTO III Investigators. A comparison of reteplase with alteplase for acute myocardial infarction. *N Engl J Med*. 1997;337:1118–1123.

23. ASSENT-2 Investigators. Single-bolus tenecteplase compared with front-loaded alteplase in acute myocardial infarction: The ASSENT-2 double-blind randomised trial. *Lancet.* 1999;354:716–722.
24. Armstrong PW, Collen D. Fibrinolysis for acute myocardial infarction: Current status and new horizons for pharmacological reperfusion, Part 1. *Circulation.* 2001;103:2862–2866.
25. Cannon CP, Gibson CM, McCabe CH, et al. TNK – tissue plasminogen activator compared with front-loaded alteplase in acute myocardial infarction: results of the TIMI 10B. *Circulation.* 1998;2805–2814.
26. Neuhaus KL, Von Essen R, Tebbe U, et al. Improved thrombolysis in acute myocardial infarction with front-loaded administration of alteplase: Results of the RT-PA-APSAC patency study (TAPS). *J Am Coll Cardiol.* 1992;19:885–891.
27. Ohman EM, Califf RM, Topol EF, et al. Consequences of reocclusion after successful reperfusion therapy in acute myocardial infarction. TAMI Study Group. *Circulation.* 1990;82:781–791.
28. D'Souza SP, Mamas MA, Fraser DG, Fath-Ordoubadi F. Routine early coronary angioplasty versus ischaemia-guided angioplasty after thrombolysis in acute ST-elevation myocardial infarction: a meta-analysis. *Eur Heart J.* 2011;32:972–982.
29. Grines CL, Browne KF, Marco J, et al. A comparison of immediate angioplasty with thrombolytic therapy in acute myocardial infarction. *N Engl J Med.* 1993;328:673–679.
30. Vogt A, Von Essen R, Tebbe U, et al. Impact of early perfusion status of the infarct-related artery on short-term mortality after thrombolysis for acute myocardial infarction: Retrospective analysis of four German multicenter studies. *J Am Coll Cardiol.* 1993;21:1391–1395.
31. Antman EM, Anbe DT, Armstrong PW, et al. ACC/AHA guidelines for the management of patients with ST-elevation myocardial infarction—executive summary. *J Am Coll Cardiol.* 2004;44:671–719.
32. Prendergast BD, Shandall A, Buchalter MB. What do we do when thrombolysis fails? A United Kingdom survey. *Int J Card.* 1997;61:39–42.
33. Gruppo Italiano per lo Studio della Sopravvivenza nell'Infarto Miocardico. GISSI-2: afactorial randomized trial of alteplase versus streptokinase and heparin versus no heparin among 12,490 patients with acute myocardial infarction. *Lancet.* 1990;336:65–71.
34. Grines CL, Booth DC, Nissen SE. Mechanism of acute myocardial infarction in patients with prior coronary artery bypass grafting and therapeutic implications. *Am J Cardiol.* 1999;65:1292–1296.
35. Sutton AGC, Campbell PG, Graham R, et al. A randomized trial of rescue angioplasty versus a conservative approach for failed fibrinolysis in ST-segment elevation myocardial infarction. *J Am Coll Cardiol.* 2004;44:287–296.

36. Sutton AGC, Campbell PG, Graham R, et al. One year results of the Middles brough early revascularisation to limit infarction (MERLIN) trial. *Heart.* 2004;91:1330–1337.
37. Gershlick AH, Stephens-Lloyd A, Hughes S, et al. Rescue angioplasty after failed thrombolytic therapy for acute myocardial infarction. *N Engl J Med.* 2005;353:2758–2768.
38. Wijeysundera HC, Vijayaraghavan R, Nallamothu BK, et al. Rescue angioplasty or repeat fibrinolysis after failed fibrinolytic therapy for ST-Segment myocardial infarction. *J Am Coll Cardiol.* 2007;49:422–430.
39. Fernandez-Aviles F, Alonso JJ, Castro-Beiras A, et al. Routine invasive strategy within 24 hours of thrombolysis versus ischaemia-guided conservative approach for acute myocardial infarction with ST-segment elevation (GRACIA-1): A randomised controlled trial. *Lancet.* 2004;364:1045–1053.
40. Le May MR, Wells GA, Labinaz M, et al. Combined angioplasty and pharmacological intervention versus thrombolysis alone in acute myocardial infarction (CAPITAL AMI study). *J Am Coll Cardiol.* 2005;46:417–424.
41. Vermeer F, Oude Ophuis AJM, Berg EJ, et al. Prospective randomized comparison between thrombolysis, rescue PTCA, and primary PTCA in patients with extensive myocardial infarction admitted to a hospital without PTCA facilities: A safety and feasibility study. *Heart.* 1999;82:426–431.
42. Widimsky P, Groch L, Zelizko M, et al. Multicentre randomized trial comparing transport to primary angioplasty vs immediate thrombolysis vs combined strategy for patients with acute myocardial infarction presenting to a community hospital without a catheterization laboratory. *Eur Heart J.* 2000;21:823–831.
43. Herrmann HC, Moliterno DJ, Ohman EM, et al. Facilitation of early percutaneous coronary intervention after reteplase with or without abciximab in acute myocardial infarction results from the SPEED (GUSTO-4 Pilot) trial. *J Am Coll Cardiol.* 2000;36:1489–1496.
44. Schweiger MJ, Cannon CP, Murphy SA, et al. Early coronary intervention following pharmacologic therapy for acute myocardial infarction (The Combined TIMI 10B–TIMI 14 Experience). *Am J Cardiol.* 2001;88:831–836.
45. Scheller B, Hennen B, Hammer B, et al. Beneficial effects of immediate stenting after thrombolysis in acute myocardial infarction. *J Am Coll Cardiol.* 2003;42:634–641.
46. Kurihara H, Matsumoto S, Tamura R, et al. Clinical outcome of percutaneous coronary intervention with antecedent mutant t-PA administration for acute myocardial infarction. *Am Heart J.* 2004;147:e14.
47. Mockel M, Bocksch W, Strohm S. Facilitated percutaneous coronary intervention (PCI) inpatients with acute ST-elevation myocardial

infarction: Comparison of prehospital tirofiban versus fibrinolysis before direct PCI. *Int J Cardiology*. 2005;103:193–200.

48. ASSENT-4 PCI Investigators. Primary versus tenecteplase-facilitated percutaneous coronary intervention in patients with ST-segment elevation acute myocardial infarction (ASSENT-4 PCI): randomised trial. *Lancet*. 2006;367:569–578.
49. Ross AM, Coyne KS, Reiner JS, et al. A randomized trial comparing primary angioplasty with a strategy of short-acting thrombolysis and immediate planned rescue angioplasty in acute myocardial infarction: The PACT Trial. *J Am Coll Cardiol*. 1999;34:1954–1962.
50. Dudek D, Zmudka K, Katuza GL, et al. Facilitated percutaneous coronary intervention in patients with acute myocardial infarction transferred from remote hospitals. *Am J Cardiol*. 2003;91:227–229.
51. Kastrati A, Mehilli J, Schlotterbeck K, et al. Early administration of reteplase plus abciximab vs abciximab alone in patients with acute myocardial infarction referred for percutaneous coronary intervention. *JAMA*. 2004;291:947–954.
52. Maioli M, Gallopin M, Leoncini M, et al. Facilitated primary coronary intervention with abciximab and very low dose of alteplase during off-hours compared with direct primary intervention during regular hours. *Cath Cardiovasc Interv*. 2005;65:484–491.
53. The ADVANCE MI Investigators. Facilitated percutaneous coronary intervention for acute ST-segment elevation myocardial infarction: Results from the prematurely terminated ADdressing the Value of facilitated ANgioplasty after Combination therapy or Eptifibatide monotherapy in acute Myocardial Infarction (ADVANCE MI) trial. *Am Heart J*. 2005;150:116–122.
54. Keely EC, Boura JA, Grines CL. Comparison of primary and facilitated percutaneous coronary interventions for ST-elevation myocardial infarction: quantitative review of randomised trials. *Lancet*. 2006;367:579–588.
55. Ellis SG, Tendera M, de Belder MA, et al. Facilitated PCI in patients with ST-elevation myocardial infarction. *N Engl J Med*. 2008;358:2205–2217.
56. Antman EM, Hand M, Armstrong PW, et al. 2007 Focused update of the ACC/AHA 2004 guidelines for the management of patients with ST-elevation myocardial infarction. *J Am Coll Cardiol*. 2008;51:210–250.
57. Di Mario C, Dudek D, Piscione F, et al. Immediate angioplasty versus standard therapy with rescue angioplasty after thrombolysis in the Combined Abciximab REteplase Stent Study in Acute Myocardial Infarction (CARESS-in-AMI): An open, prospective, randomised, multicentre trial. *Lancet*. 2008;371:559–568.
58. Cantor WJ, Fitchett D, Borgundvaag B, et al. Routine early angioplasty after fibrinolysis for acute myocardial infarction. *N Engl J Med*. 2009;360:2705–2718.

59. Bohmer E, Hoffmann P, Abdelnoor M, et al. Thrombolysis in acute myocardial infarction in areas with very long transfer distances results of the NORDISTEMI (Norwegian study on district treatment of ST-elevation myocardial infarction). *J Am Coll Cardiol.* 2010;55:102–110.
60. Wijeysundera HC, You JJ, Nallamothu BK, et al. An early invasive strategy versus ischemia-guided management after fibrinolytic therapy for ST-segment elevation myocardial infarction: A meta-analysis of contemporary randomized controlled trials. *Am Heart J.* 2008;156:564.e2–572.e2.
61. Stenestrand U, Lindback J, Wallentin L, et al. Long-term outcome of primary percutaneous coronary intervention vs prehospital and in-hospital thrombolysis for patients with ST-elevation myocardial infarction. *JAMA.* 2006;296:1749–1756.
62. Pinto DS, Kirtane AJ, Nallamothu BK, et al. Hospital delays in reperfusion for ST-elevation myocardial infarction: Implications when selecting a reperfusion strategy. *Circulation.* 2006;114:2019–2025.
63. Leon MB, Baim DS, Popma JJ, et al. A clinical trial comparing three antithrombotic-drug regimens after coronary-artery stenting. stent anticoagulation restenosis study investigators. *N Engl J Med.* 1998;339:1665–1671.
64. Mehta SR, Tanguay JF, Eikelboom JW, et al. Double-dose versus standard-dose clopidogrel and high-dose versus low-dose aspirin in individuals undergoing percutaneous coronary intervention for acute coronary syndromes (CURRENT-OASIS 7): A randomised factorial trial. *Lancet.* 2010;376:1233–1243.
65. Mehta SR, Bassand JP, et al. Dose comparisons of clopidogrel and aspirin in acute coronary syndromes. *N Engl J Med.* 2010;363:930–942.
66. Wiviott SD, Braunwald E, McCabe CH, et al. Prasugrel versus clopidogrel in patients with acute coronary syndromes. *N Engl J Med.* 2007;357:2001–2015.
67. Held C, Asenblad N, Bassand JP, et al. Ticagrelor versus clopidogrel in patients with acute coronary syndromes undergoing coronary artery bypass surgery: Results from the PLATO (platelet inhibition and patient outcomes) trial. *J Am Coll Cardiol.* 2011;57:672–684.
68. De Luca G, Suryapranata H, Stone GW, et al. Abciximab as adjunctive therapy to reperfusion in acute ST-segment elevation myocardial infarction: A meta-analysis of randomized trials. *JAMA.* 2005;293:1759–1765.
69. Van't Hof AW, Ten Berg J, Heestermans T, et al. Prehospital initiation of tirofiban in patients with ST-elevation myocardial infarction undergoing primary angioplasty (on-TIME 2): A multicentre, double-blind, randomised controlled trial. *Lancet.* 2008;372:537–546.
70. Montalescot G, Barragan P, Wittenberg O, et al. Platelet glycoprotein IIb/IIIa inhibition with coronary stenting for acute myocardial infarction. *N Engl J Med.*2001;344:1895–1903.

71. Mehilli J, Kastrati A, Schulz S, et al. Abciximab in patients with acute ST-segment-elevation myocardial infarction undergoing primary percutaneous coronary intervention after clopidogrel loading: a randomized double-blind trial. *Circulation*. 2009;119:1933–1940.
72. Bonnefoy E, Lapostolle F, Leizorovicz A, et al. Primary angioplasty versus prehospital fibrinolysis in acute myocardial infarction: A randomised study. *Lancet*. 2002;360:825–829.
73. Bonnefoy E, Steg PG, Boutitie F, et al. Comparison of primary angioplasty and pre-hospital fibrinolysis in acute myocardial infarction (CAPTIM) trial: A 5-year follow-up. *Eur Heart J*.2009;30:1598–1606.
74. Armstrong PW. A comparison of pharmacologic therapy with/without timely coronary intervention vs. primary percutaneous intervention early after ST-elevation myocardial infarction: the WEST (Which Early ST-elevation myocardial infarction Therapy) study. *Eur Heart J*. 2006;27:1530–1538.
75. Come PC, Pitt B. Nitroglycerin-induced severe hypotension and bradycardia in patients with acute myocardial infarction. *Circulation*. 1976;54:624–628.
76. Moradkhan R, Sinoway LI. Revisiting the role of oxygen therapy in cardiac patients. *J Am Coll Cardiol*. 2010;56:1013–1016.
77. McNulty PH, King N, Scott S, et al. Effects of supplemental oxygen administration on coronary blood flow in patients undergoing cardiac catheterization. *Am J Physiol Heart Circ Physiol*. 2005;288:H1057–H1062.
78. Wallentin L, Goldstein P, Armstrong PW, et al. Efficacy and safety of tenecteplase in combination with the low-molecular-weight heparin enoxaparin or unfractionated heparin in the prehospital setting: The assessment of the safety and efficacy of a new thrombolytic regimen (ASSENT)-3 PLUS randomized trial in acute myocardial infarction. *Circulation*. 2003;108:135–142.
79. Antman EM, Morrow DA, McCabe CH, et al. Enoxaparin versus unfractionated heparin with fibrinolysis for ST-elevation myocardial infarction. *N Engl J Med*. 2006;354:1477–1488.
80. Montalescot G, Zeymer U, Silvain J, et al. Intravenous enoxaparin or unfractionated heparin in primary percutaneous coronary intervention for ST-elevation myocardial infarction: The international randomised open-label ATOLL trial. *Lancet*. 2011;378:693–703.
81. Armstrong PW, Gershlick AH, Goldstein P, et al. STREAM Investigative Team. Fibrinolysis or primary PCI in ST-segment elevation myocardial infarction. *N Engl J Med*. 2013;368:1379–1387.

CHAPTER 3

Prehospital ECG Acquisition/ Interpretation: Emerging Technology Applied to STEMI Care

Michael J. Pompliano, BS, EMT, and
George L. Adams, MD, MHS

INTRODUCTION

Effectiveness of emergency management for STEMI relies on the speed and accuracy of symptom identification, diagnosis, and appropriate triage. Electrocardiography is the gold standard for the diagnosis of STEMI and is the central tool in systems of STEMI care for both prehospital and hospital settings.

Prehospital transmission of ECGs has revolutionized STEMI systems of care by mobilizing resources and assisting healthcare professionals to decide on a plan of care before the patient reaches the hospital. Examples include: (1) thrombolytics are given by paramedics in the field for STEMI patients whose transmitted ECG has been confirmed by an emergency medical physician; (2) confirmation of an STEMI through a transmitted ECG may result in paramedics bypassing a hospital for another to receive primary percutaneous coronary intervention (PPCI) treatment; (3) transmitted ECGs allow a treating cardiologist and

Prehospital Management of Acute STEMI: Practical Approaches and International Strategies for Early Intervention © 2015 Joseph S. Alpert, Lynne T. Braun, Barbara J. Fletcher, Gerald Fletcher, Editors-in-Chief, Cardiotext Publishing, ISBN: 978-1-935395-66-9

the catheterization staff to be mobilized in off hours before the patient reaches the hospital to expedite care (staff arrive before the patient and able to pull equipment on the basis of ECG to expedite care). Each one of these scenarios increases the time to treatment, resulting in a reduction in morbidity and mortality.

However, current research shows prehospital ECGs are only used in 10% to 25% of patients with STEMI, despite a survey which showed 90.6% of emergency medical services (EMS) systems serving the 200 largest U.S. cities had 12-lead ECG equipment available in their ambulance systems.[1,2] Thus, even though the equipment is available, it is largely underutilized. An effective strategy for improving systems of care for STEMI patients would implement prehospital 12-lead electrocardiography programs that incorporate the input of a cardiologist and cardiac care team as early as possible in diagnosis and triage decision making of STEMI patients.[3-5] This chapter will discuss some of the technological advances that make it easier to obtain accurate ECG tracings and coordinate diagnostic capabilities.

ADVANCEMENTS IN TECHNOLOGY

Prehospital ECGs have the potential to significantly improve the diagnostic accuracy in chest pain patients and assist in triage. Technological advancements, specifically telemedicine, allow for wireless transmission of ECGs by using a cellular connection or a digital wireless network. This greatly increases the opportunity for physician input for diagnosis and treatment decisions in the field before arrival to the hospital. The available technology allows individual communities to utilize preconfigured Bluetooth devices, preprogrammed receiving and transmitting stations, dedicated e-mail servers, and smartphones to develop fully automated wireless networks and available resources specific to their community needs. These fully automated wireless networks are capable of facilitating simultaneous 12-lead ECG transmission from EMS personnel in the field to the Emergency Department (ED) and offsite cardiologists via receiving station and smartphone, respectively.

Another benefit from advanced technology is the ability to acquire serial ECGs. Even under optimal circumstances, some STEMI cases may not meet diagnostic criteria on prehospital ECGs. If prehospital ECGs show questionable findings that may potentially result in a developed ST-segment elevation, serial ECGs may assist in patient monitoring. Initial timing of the ECG may be misleading depending on the time it is obtained during the symptom onset. If obtained early in the symptom complex, the patient may be inappropriately triaged.[6] Serial ECGs allow the physician to see changes over multiple ECGs, increasing diagnostic accuracy as a result. Studies have shown serial ECG sensitivities of 90% and specificities of 98%, compared with 76% and 98% without serial ECGs.[7] Verbeek et al.[9] retrospectively analyzed 325 consecutive prehospital STEMIs.[8] If the first ECG did not identify STEMI, protocol required a second ECG just before transport and, if necessary, a third ECG before entering the receiving ED. STEMI was identified on the first prehospital ECG in 275 cases (84.6%), on the second ECG in 30 cases (93.8%), and on the third ECG in 20 cases (100%). For STEMIs identified on the second or third ECG, 90% were identified within 25 minutes after the first ECG; this finding suggest that serial ECGs taken en route to the hospital utilize transport time much more efficiently.[6] In hindsight, a single prehospital ECG would have identified only 84.6% of STEMI patients, which suggests caution is warranted in using a single prehospital ECG to rule out STEMI. [9]

ECG ACQUISITION

Prehospital 12-lead electrocardiography acquisition involves multiple steps, including application of recording electrodes, capture of electrocardiographic data, automated interpretation by using diagnostic algorithms within the device, transmission capabilities, and the option for over-read of the output by EMS personnel.[10]

Studies have shown that the time for acquisition of the prehospital ECG does not delay transport. Prehospital ECGs may be obtained within 2 minutes and can save a considerable amount of time for definitive care, once the patient arrives at the receiving facility.[11] Prehospital ECGs may be acquired on-scene without unwarranted delay in patient transport, provide comparable data quality to ECGs obtained in a hospital setting, and provide the ED with a comparison of previously performed ECGs as well as a tracing to compare with the ECG that will be performed within minutes after the patient's ED arrival.[11,12]

Lead Misplacement

Although ECGs have proven to be useful tools in the diagnosis and triage of STEMI patients, inaccurate STEMI diagnosis or inappropriate triage may evolve from inaccurate ECG interpretations, potentially prompting EMS personnel to withhold necessary therapy or administer unnecessary therapy.[13] A common cause of inaccurate ECG trace interpretation is improper acquisition from electrode misplacement; studies have shown 17% to 24% of patients were given a different diagnosis when the 12-lead ECG was acquired using the incorrect electrode configuration, and 11% had STEMI diagnosis due to incorrect electrode configuration.[13] These findings highlight the importance of further educating medical and paramedical personnel regarding ECG acquisition.

INTERPRETATION ACCURACY

After timely acquisition of a prehospital ECG, the next important step is accurate interpretation and diagnosis. The three basic options for prehospital ECG interpretation are automated systems, paramedics, and physicians. Often all three are used together, and an automated ECG interpretation is over-read by trained personnel.

Automated ECG Interpretation

Automated ECG interpretation is the use of diagnostic algorithms within the device to analyze ECG tracing results for the presence of identifiable patterns that indicate different ischemic events. Individual algorithms are capable of obtaining precise measurements, detecting abnormal variations, and producing simplified results to be reviewed by the ECG operator. In addition, algorithms can provide a quality score that indicates the presence of technical problems with the tracing itself. ECG quality algorithms help inexperienced nurses and paramedics interpret diagnostic-quality ECGs with >90% accuracy by detecting microscopic errors and providing a quality score to the user.[14]

With the proper acquisition of a prehospital ECG, automated ECG interpretation algorithms have shown high degrees of accuracy and have proven to be an effective tool for patient triage, especially in the absence of a cardiologist's interpretation.[15] However, the automated ECG interpretation algorithms are not without limitations. Inaccuracies in automated ECG interpretation may result from movement artifact, lead misplacement, or poor skin contact, resulting in a poor-quality tracing that can be misinterpreted by algorithms or EMS providers.[4] Additionally, algorithms can provide a quality score that indicates the presence of technical problems with the tracing itself. Although accurate automated interpretation depends largely on the correct acquisition of an ECG, interpretation accuracy may further be limited by large individual variations in coronary anatomy, preexisting conditions, collateral circulation, and confounders, or technical shortcomings in detecting electrical impulses from certain regions of the heart.[16]

Results vary when comparing the accuracy of automated ECG interpretation with that of physician electrocardiographers.

Kudenchuk et al.[17] investigated the accuracy of computer-interpreted ECGs, in which a standard 12-lead ECG was obtained by paramedics for 1189 suspected STEMI patients via a battery-powered ECG that had both computer-interpretive and cellular telephone transmission capabilities. The electrocardiographer proved to have a higher sensitivity (66%), using less stringent diagnostic criteria, compared with the computer-interpreted ECG (52%); however, the automated interpretation specificity was 98% compared with the 95% specificity of the electrocardiographer.

Clinical variables also have an impact on the ECG accuracy. Kudenchuk et al.[17] noted that the sensitivity of both the computer and electrocardiographer interpretations significantly improved when younger patients, particularly those without prior cardiac disease (AMI, angina, or CHF), were evaluated.[17] The correct diagnosis was similarly affected by STEMI location—anterior STEMIs, which were equally common between patients with and without AMI, produced a computer-interpretation sensitivity of 56%; whereas inferior STEMIs, which were almost always associated with acute infarction, resulted in a computer-interpretation sensitivity of 87%.[17]

Because of these limitations, most regions that use prehospital ECGs have standard protocols that govern what types of symptoms should prompt acquisition of an ECG trace, but the false-positive and false-negative rates of ECG interpretation have been poorly characterized in general.[4] A complete review of ischemic versus nonischemic ST elevation patterns on the ECG is available in the next chapter.

Paramedic Education and ECG Interpretation

Current national EMS education standards include 12-lead ECG interpretation and continuous ECG monitoring as a required competency for paramedics. Similarly, paramedics are the most common source of prehospital ECG acquisition and supply emergency management systems with the first and most convenient opportunity for human interpretation of ECG tracings.[18] However, no current standards exist for the initial or continuing education requirements to achieve and maintain competency in prehospital ECG interpretation. Standards are also needed for protocols to obtain an ECG for certain patient subsets and to develop triage criteria in these situations. The lack of clear standards does allow more flexibility for smaller communities and rural areas to design systems that most efficiently use their available resources. Simultaneously, the lack of standards might have a negative impact on the diagnostic accuracy.

Le May et al.[19] sought to determine whether advanced care paramedics (ACPs) could accurately identify STEMI on the prehospital ECG and contribute to strategies that shorten the time to reperfusion.[19] The ACPs' results for identifying STEMI on the ECG showed a sensitivity of 95%, a specificity of 96%, a positive predictive value of 82%, and a negative predictive value of 99%.

Physician ECG interpretation

With the modern advanced wireless transmission capabilities, it is possible to receive real-time remote interpretation of prehospital 12-lead ECGs by expert physician electrocardiographers.[20] For the ED physicians or on-call cardiologists to interpret a prehospital ECG recorded in the field, it must first be wirelessly transmitted to a receiving center in the ED or the on-call cardiologist's cell phone. A study has previously shown that the cardiologists' decisions did not vary significantly when viewing either traditional paper ECGs or LCD screen ECGs.[21] Physicians have historically shown high accuracies in the interpretations of prehospital ECGs. In one such study (861 ECGs over 12 months), physicians were able to obtain 90% sensitivity and 94% specificity when identifying ECG STEMIs, compared with EMS accuracy of 71% sensitivity and 97% specificity for STEMI diagnosis.[22] In addition, the rates of inappropriate thrombolysis given by EMS, on the basis of prehospital ECG interpretation, have been reported to be approximately 3.2%, compared with a rate of 1.9% on the basis of physician diagnosis.[23]

BENEFITS OF ECG TELEMEDICINE FOR TRIAGE AND MOBILIZATION OF RESOURCES

A STEMI system depends on the recognition of a STEMI by prehospital care providers, usually through the acquisition and interpretation of a prehospital ECG. Telemedicine provides a means for coordinating diagnostic skills and triage decisions throughout the entire STEMI prehospital care system.

Triage

One of the most significant benefits is the utilization of wireless prehospital ECGs during the triage of suspected-STEMI patients. With accurate identification of STEMI from prehospital ECGs, EMS personnel can bypass the local ED and transport STEMI patients directly to the cardiac catheterization suite of a PPCI center; this has increased the proportion of patients for whom first medical contact to balloon inflation time was <90 minutes from 28.4% to 91.3%.[8] With STEMI identification from prehospital ECGs rapidly becoming a point of focus for streamlining STEMI care, more attention has been given to ECG interpretation accuracy.

A study comparing paramedic prehospital triage without transmission of the ECG, in which all paramedics received an additional 4 hours of training on 12-lead ECG for identification of STEMI, found 90% agreement with physician triage according to interpretation of ECG. Patients with suspected STEMI on the prehospital ECG bypassed the closest hospital for emergent coronary angiography and PPCI, and the median first medical contact to balloon time was 91 minutes. Cantor et al.[24] concluded that STEMI patients can be safely and effectively transported directly for PPCI by paramedics without advanced care training. In support of their conclusion, other studies have shown that training paramedics to recognize STEMI on a 12-lead ECG is feasible and suggest that radio transmission may not be necessary to prealert the hospital.[25]

Dhruva et al.[26] enrolled 80 patients with successful prehospital ECG transmission via wireless cellular phone network reducing door-to-intervention time to 80.1 minutes, compared with 145.6 minutes in the year before. Median time from prehospital ECG acquisition to availability on the remote server was 2 minutes and on the smartphone was 4 minutes. The Timely Intervention in Myocardial Emergency, North-East (TIME-NE) trial[3] instituted a STEMI system by utilizing prehospital cellular ECG transmission directly to a cardiologist's handheld device. The median door-to-reperfusion time for patients with successful electrocardiographic transmission was 50 minutes, which was significantly shorter than preintervention EMS transport without ECG transmission of 101 minutes ($P < 0.0001$).

In addition to accurate interpretations, cardiologists have been able to effectively use automated ECG interpretation programs as triage tools to assist in triage decision making.[15] The study findings suggest that automated ECG interpretation programs are a reliable indication for triage in the absence of an on-call cardiologist. Regardless, the ECG tracing itself, not the automated report, was still the dominant factor in the decision-making process.[15]

Mobilization of Resources

If patients are evaluated in the ED, the evaluation should be streamlined having a physician and necessary resources (e.g., translators, nurses) ready before patient arrival, following a standard protocol for treatment and minimizing physical movement, such as transferring between stretchers. In a study of a system involving ECG transmission, transmission was successful in 89% of attempts, with most failures due to human error, including forgetting to recharge batteries and carry the phone when on call; Sillesen et al.[27] concluded it was reasonable to assume that such errors could be minimized in the future by adhering to a stricter protocol and routines. The study showed a 7-minute increase in on-scene time after implementation of the prehospital ECG recording, but noted that the lost time in the prehospital setting was won back in the hospital, because early notification of the catheterization suite personnel allowed the catheterization suite to be operational upon patient arrival (Figure 3.1).[27] Of the 27 patients referred directly for PPCI, the median door-to-PPCI time was 22 minutes, a reduction of 72 minutes compared with historic controls. In addition, patients referred during regular hours were delayed 12 minutes shorter than for patients redirected during off-hours, which may support the feasibility of turning conventional PCI centers into "24/7 on-call" centers. Sillesen et al.[27] concluded that prehospital ECG assisted in patient triage, resulting in reduced delays for PPCI treatment.

In an urban area, it is possible to utilize new technology that allows transmission of prehospital ECG to a handheld device carried by the attending cardiologist for immediate ECG evaluation, irrespective of physical location. Twelve-lead prehospital ECG transmission directly to a cardiologist's

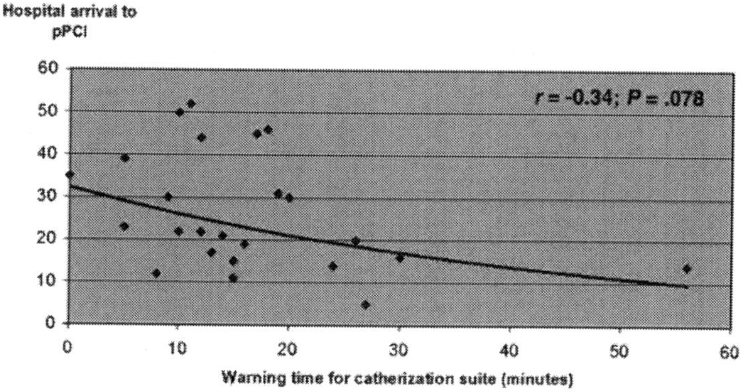

Figure 3.1

Early activation of the cardiac catheterization suite.[27] With permission from Elsevier.

mobile telephone with immediate triage and referral of patients with STEMI directly to a catheterization suite was extremely efficient, allowing EMS to bypass local hospitals and decreasing door-to-PCI time by more than an hour. With successful transmission in 94% of attempted patients, PCI was initiated within 90 minutes after the 911 calls in 72% of patients, versus 18% of patients in the control group.[28]

Cardiac Catheterization Laboratory Activation

In recent years, PPCI has begun to play a larger role in the management of STEMI because of the growing push for rapid and effective reperfusion. Thus, the prehospital activation of the cardiac catheterization lab (CCL) based on prehospital ECG is also becoming a cornerstone of therapy in many large centers.[23] Prior to the activation of the CCL, it is necessary for prehospital personnel to efficiently differentiate the smaller acute-STEMI cohort from the larger "chest pain" cohort; false activations of the CCL resulting from inaccuracies during ECG interpretation or triage decision making can be very costly to the system. Recent studies have highlighted distinctions between inappropriate and false activations, defining false activations with respect to a patient's final diagnosis of STEMI.[29] These false activations, which may be as high as 28%, were associated with inappropriate activation rates of 13% according to ECG criteria, further highlighting the significant impact of confounders and other factors.[29] Current strategies and recommendations related to this issue are discussed further in Chapter 5.

FUTURE OF THE PREHOSPITAL ECG AND TELEMEDICINE

Historically, paramedics' ability to read ECGs has been poor. With the technology to assist in interpretation and transmission of ECGs, and the interprofessional team's motivation to train them, paramedics have an important role in the emergency STEMI response system (Figure 3.2).[30] Empowering them to read and transmit ECGs to activate the team-based response faster has proven to positively influence the outcome of the patient. This technology is not limited to STEMI patients, and can be applied to other things (e.g., stroke, etc.) in the prehospital setting.

Although the positive contributions of prehospital ECGs and telemedicine to patient outcomes have been investigated and well documented, this technology continues to be underutilized because of various barriers to the implementation of prehospital ECG programs, such as the costs of device acquisition and replacement, paramedic training, and ongoing competency assessment. Integrated devices currently cost around US$9000 to $25,000 each, but the cost of equipment is likely to decrease in the future as it becomes the standard of care.[10] Other barriers to implementing systems are more

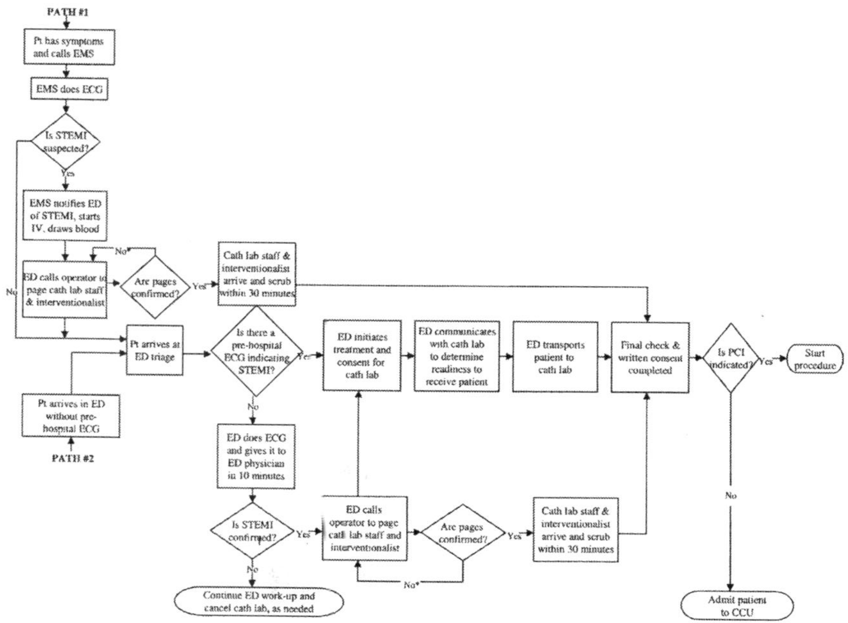

Figure 3.2

Flow chart of the emergency STEMI response system.[30] With permission from Elsevier.

logistics-based, especially in smaller communities with limited resources or rural areas that lack the capability to efficiently train their personnel; as such, authority and funding for these programs may need to come from higher levels of government, such as county, state, or regional health agencies.[4] In addition, many systems include several for-profit EMS agencies that are responsible for evaluating and transporting patients, which may necessitate that prehospital ECGs are required by regulation and are reimbursed. Successful 12-lead ECG programs use technology as a tool to create a seamless community of care between the prehospital and hospital environments.[31]

CONCLUSION

Models of prehospital patient assessment, triage, and identification of suspected STEMI vary by jurisdiction but are contingent upon accurate prehospital ECG interpretation and optimal communication between EMS and reperfusion facilities. Successful emergency response systems desire a test that is both sensitive enough to avoid missing an opportunity for life-saving treatment and specific enough to minimize false activation of the CCL and inappropriate thrombolysis.[23] The point at which sensitivity is sacrificed for specificity is not known, nor is there a clear guide available to define the acceptable levels of false positives and negatives. However, the available data has shown that prehospital ECG interpretation, via EMS or ECG transmission, is safe, reliable, and plays a pivotal role in the care of STEMI patients. As such, prehospital ECG interpretation, regardless of the method used, should be the standard of care for chest pain presentations.

REFERENCES

1. Williams DM. 200-city survey: EMS from all angles. *JEMS*. 2008;1.
2. Diercks DB, Kontos MC, Chen AY, et al. Utilization and impact of prehospital electrocardiograms for patients with acute ST-segment elevation myocardial infarction: Data from the NCDR (National

Cardiovascular Data Registry) ACTION (Acute Coronary Treatment and Intervention Outcomes Network) Registry. *J Am Coll Cardiol.* 2009;53(2):161–166.

3. Cambell PT, Patterson J, Cromer D, et al. Prehospital triage of acute myocardial infarction: Wireless transmission of electrocardiograms to the on-call cardiologist via a handheld computer. *J Electrocardiol.* 2005;38(4):300–309.
4. Ting HH, Krumholz HM, Bradley EH, et al. Implementation and integration of prehospital ECGs into systems of care for acute coronary syndrome: A scientific statement from the American Heart Association Interdisciplinary Council on Quality of Care and Outcomes Research, Emergency Cardiovascular Care Committee, Council on Cardiovascular Nursing, and Council on Clinical Cardiology. *Circulation.* 2008;118(10):1066–1079.
5. Antman EM, Hand M, Armstrong PW, et al. 2007 focused update of the ACC/AHA 2004 guidelines for the management of patients with ST-elevation myocardial infarction. *Circulation.* 2008;117:296–329.
6. Kudenchuk PJ, Maynard C, Cobb LA, et al. Utility of the prehospital electrocardiogram in diagnosing acute coronary syndromes: The Myocardial Infarction Triage and Intervention (MITI) Project. *J Am Coll Cardiol.* 1998;32(1)17–27.
7. Gregg RE, Deluca DC, Chien CH, et al. Automated serial ECG comparison improves computerized interpretation of 12-lead ECG. *J Electrocardiol.* 2012;45(6):561–565.
8. Cheskes S, Turner L, Foggett R, et al. Paramedic contact to balloon in less than 90 minutes: A successful strategy for ST-segment elevation myocardial infarction bypass to primary percutaneous coronary intervention in a Canadian emergency medical system. *Prehosp Emerg Care.* 2011;15(4):490–498.
9. Verbeek PR, Ryan D, Turner L, et al. Serial prehospital 12-lead electrocardiograms increase identification of ST-segment elevation myocardial infarction. *Prehosp Emerg Care.* 2012;16(1):109–114.
10. Garvey JL, MacLeod BA, Sopko G, et al. Pre-Hospital 12-Lead Electrocardiography Programs: A call for implementation by emergency medical services systems providing advanced life support. *J Am Coll Cardiol.* 2006;47(3):485–491.
11. Slovis CM. The importance of prehospital ECGs. *JEMS.* 2006;31(7):S5-S6.
12. Grim P, Feldman T, Martin M, et al. Cellular telephone transmission of 12-lead electrocardiograms from ambulance to hospital. *Am J Cardiol.* 1987;60:715–720.
13. Bond RR, Finlay DD, Nugent CD, et al. The effects of electrode misplacement on clinicians' interpretation of the standard 12-lead electrocardiogram. *Eur J Intern Med.* 2012;23(7):610–615.

14. Johannesen L, Galeotti L. Automatic ECG quality scoring methodology: mimicking human annotators. *Physiol Meas.* 2012;33(9):1479–1489.
15. Clark EN, Sejersten M, Clemmensen P, et al. Automated electrocardiogram interpretation programs versus cardiologists' triage decision making based on teletransmitted data in patients with suspected acute coronary syndrome. *Am J Cardiol.* 2010;106(12):1696–1702.
16. Rokos IC, French WJ, Mattu A, et al. Appropriate cardiac cath lab activation: Optimizing electrocardiogram interpretation and clinical decision-making for acute ST-elevation myocardial infarction. *Am Heart J.* 2010;160(6):995–1003.
17. Kudenchuk PJ, Ho MT, Weaver WD, et al. Accuracy of computer interpreted electrocardiography in selecting patients for thrombolytic therapy. *J Am Coll Cardiol.* 1991;17(7):1486–1491.
18. US Department of Transportation: National Highway Traffic Safety Administration. National Emergency Medical Services Education Standards. January 2009. Available at: www.ems.gov.
19. Le May MR, Dionne R, Maloney J, et al. Diagnostic performance and potential clinical impact of advanced care paramedic interpretation of ST-segment elevation myocardial infarction in the field. *CJEM.* 2006;8(6):401–407.
20. Terkelsen CJ, Norgaard BL, Lassen JF, et al. Telemedicine used for remote prehospital diagnosing in patients suspected of acute myocardial infarction. *J Intern Med.* 2002;252(5):412–420.
21. Leibrandt PN, Bell SJ, Savona MR, et al. Validation of cardiologists' decisions to initiate reperfusion therapy for acute myocardial infarction with electrocardiograms viewed on liquid crystal displays of cellular telephones. *Am Heart J.* 2000;140(5):747–752.
22. Keeling P, Hughes D, Price L, et al. Safety and feasibility of prehospital thrombolysis carried out by paramedics. *BMJ.* 2003;327(7405)27–28.
23. Ducas RA, Wassef AW, Jassal DS, et al. To transmit or not to transmit: how good are emergency medical personnel in detecting STEMI in patients with chest pain? *Can J Cardiol.* 2012;28(4):432–437.
24. Cantor WJ, Hoogeveen P, Robert A, et al. Prehospital diagnosis and triage of ST-elevation myocardial infarction by paramedics without advanced care training. *Am Heart J.* 2012;164(2):201–206.
25. Whitbread M, Leah V, Bell T, et al. Recognition of ST elevation by paramedics. *Emerg Med J.* 2002;19(1):66–67.
26. Dhruva VN, Abdelhadi SI, Anis A, et al. ST-segment analysis using wireless technology in acute myocardial infarction (STAT-MI) trial. *J Am Coll Cardiol.* 2007;50(6):509–513.
27. Sillesen M, Sejersten M, Strange S, et al. Referral of patients with ST-segment elevation acute myocardial infarction directly to the catheterization suite based on prehospital teletransmission of 12-lead electrocardiogram. *J Electrocardiol.* 2008;41(1)49–53.

28. Sejersten M, Sillesen M, Hansen PR, et al. Effect on treatment delay of prehospital teletransmission of 12-lead electrocardiogram to a cardiologist for immediate triage and direct referral of patients. *Am J Cardiol.* 2008;101(7):941–946.
29. Mixon TA, Suhr E, Caldwell G, et al. Retrospective description and analysis of consecutive catheterization laboratory ST-segment elevation myocardial infarction activations with proposal, rationale, and use of a new classification scheme. *Circ Cardiovasc Qual Outcomes.* 2012;5;62–59.
30. Bradley EH, Roumanis SA, Radford MJ, et al. Achieving door-to-balloon times that meet quality guidelines. How do successful hospitals do it? *J Am Coll Cardiol.* 2005;46(7):1236–1241.
31. McCallion T. Applying – not just implementing – a 12-lead program. *JEMS.* 2006;31(7):S13–S22.

CHAPTER 4

ECG Pitfalls in Early Recognition of STEMI: Ischemic Versus Nonischemic ST Elevation

Henry D. Huang, MD, Waleed Kayani, MD, Salman Bandeali, MD, and Yochai Birnbaum, MD

INTRODUCTION

The guidelines for ST-elevation myocardial infarction (STEMI) recommend immediate reperfusion therapy in patients reported within 12 hours of onset of symptoms compatible with myocardial infarction (even if resolved) and concomitant ST-segment elevation (STE) in 2 or more adjacent leads.[1,2] In an effort to meet these goals, the American College of Cardiology Foundation (ACCF)/American Heart Association (AHA) guidelines for STEMI recommend that ECG diagnosis of STEMI be made within 10 minutes of first medical contact in patient presenting with suspected STEMI.[2] However, not all patients with STE on their presenting ECG necessarily have transmural ischemia owing to acute thrombotic occlusion of an epicardial coronary artery; that is, a significant number of patients with nonischemic STE (NISTE) are unnecessarily exposed to the hazards of invasive procedures and medications usually reserved for STEMI.[3-6] Although cardiac troponin and creatine kinase myocardial

Prehospital Management of Acute STEMI: Practical Approaches and International Strategies for Early Intervention © 2015 Joseph S. Alpert, Lynne T. Braun, Barbara J. Fletcher, Gerald Fletcher, Editors-in-Chief, Cardiotext Publishing, ISBN: 978-1-935395-66-9

band (CK-MB) levels are useful in the diagnosis and management of non-ST elevation myocardial infarction (NSTEMI), they cannot be relied upon for diagnosis of acute STEMI in the early stages because serum levels may be undetectable for up to 6 hours following coronary artery occlusion, and decisions concerning urgent reperfusion therapy are usually made before troponin levels are detectable. Further, elderly patients, women, and patients with diabetes may present with atypical symptoms, making accurate assessment of the initial ECG even more important for decision making in these situations.[7-9] Therefore, prompt and correct interpretation of an ECG is of utmost importance.[10]

It seems that in the "real-world," the ability of physicians to differentiate NISTE from STEMI on the basis of the presenting ECG pattern widely varies. Larson et al.[11] reported that 14% of patients who were suspected to have STEMI and referred for primary percutaneous coronary intervention (PPCI) were found to have no clear culprit lesions, indicating that they had NISTE. In a study from Denmark, only 79% of the patients who were referred for direct PPCI based upon a prehospital ECG showing STE had a final diagnosis of STEMI or died.[12] Tran et al.[13] found that there were broad inconsistencies among 8 experienced interventional cardiologists practicing in a large, urban medical center when asked (1) to distinguish acute STEMI from NISTE on presenting ECGs of patients with compatible symptoms and (2) whether or not they would activate the PPCI protocol on the basis of those ECG findings.[13] Of the 84 patients with STE on their presenting ECG, 40 (48%) had adjudicated STEMI after review of their clinical records. The percentage of cases for which readers recommended PPCI varied (33%–75%). The readers' answers also varied significantly, and the sensitivity and specificity ranged from 55% to 83% (average 71%) and 32% to 86% (average 63%), respectively.[13]

It must be remembered that the differential diagnosis of STE is broad, and multiple situations warranting different approaches to treatment can present with STE on ECG, such as true acute STEMI, baseline STE without ischemia, conduction delay or ventricular pacing with secondary repolarization abnormalities, conditions with comorbid ischemia (such as aortic dissection), and conditions with new STE and chest pain but without ischemia (i.e., pericarditis or myocarditis). Table 4.1 lists common patterns of NISTE, many of which will be reviewed in detail in this chapter. Naturally, the current emphasis on diagnosing acute STEMI in a timely manner increases the pressure on all the medical personnel in contact with the potential STEMI patient and also increases the chances of overcalling "STEMI" and unnecessarily activating the catheterization laboratory or giving thrombolytics. Thus, the authors' goal in this chapter is to help readers

Table 4.1
Common patterns of NISTE

Concave STE
Normal variant of STE
Early repolarization pattern
Hypercalcemia
Hyperkalemia
Pericarditis
LVH and secondary STE
Conduction defects (LBBB and IVCD) with secondary STE
Wolff-Parkinson-White syndrome (preexcitation)
Brugada pattern
Takotsubo syndrome (apical ballooning syndrome)
Old myocardial infarction/aneurysm
Spontaneously reperfused myocardial infarction

Abbreviations: NISTE, nonischemic ST elevation; STE, ST elevation; LBBB, left bundle branch block; IVCD, intraventricular conduction delay.

in distinguishing between STEMI and NISTE on ECG by describing some of the more frequently encountered or more important causes of NISTE and illustrating some examples. It should be emphasized that the ECG should be always read in conjunction with the history and physical examination. This significantly increases the accuracy of the interpretation. It must be cautioned, however, that the patients presenting with chest pain and showing benign pattern of NISTE [e.g., "early repolarization" or STE secondary to left ventricular hypertrophy (LVH)] may have true ischemic pain and NSTEMI or even STEMI on top of their baseline benign pattern in rare instances.

PREVALENCE OF BENIGN NISTE

For the majority of healthy individuals, the ST segment is isoelectric; however, there are reports suggesting that benign NISTE is as common as 15% in the general population. Hiss et al.[14] reported that 91% of 6014 healthy men in the US Air Force who were between 16 and 58 years old had STE of 0.1 to 0.3 mV in >1 precordial leads (most commonly seen in lead V_2). Surawicz and Parikh[15] reported that the prevalence of STE >0.1 mV in one or more leads in V_1 through V_4 in 529 healthy men was 93% among those who were between 17 and 24 years old. The prevalence declined gradually with increasing age (30% in men >76 years).[15] Given that the majority of men have STE >1 mm in leads V_2-V_3, baseline STE is actually considered a normal finding rather than a variant, and is often referred to as a male pattern. Approximately 20% of women had STE >0.1 mV, and this prevalence is not affected by age.[15] Reflecting these findings, the document on "Universal Definition of Myocardial Infarction" states that the cutoffs for STEMI for leads V_2-V_3 are STE at the J-point of >0.25 mV in healthy men under the age of 40 years, >0.2 mV in men older than 40 years, and >0.15 mV in women, and/or >0.1 mV in all other leads.[16] This cutoff is reserved for patients without signs of LVH or left bundle branch block (LBBB), as patients with such ECG patterns may have marked baseline NISTE in leads V_2-V_3. Currently, there is no cutoff for NISTE for such patients.

"CONCAVE" VERSUS "CONVEX" PATTERN OF STE

The ACC/AHA guidelines suggest that it is less likely that STEMI is present if the upward-directed ST-segment changes are concave rather than convex.[1] However, Smith[17] reported that 43% of patients (16/37) who underwent emergent PPCI of the left anterior descending coronary artery had concave morphology of STE in the anterior leads, concluding that this feature was unable to exclude STEMI. This pattern is seen more frequently in the early stages of STEMI when the T waves are tall and positive. Later on, when the terminal part of the T wave becomes inverted, the ST configuration becomes convex. STEMI should not be excluded in patients with concave STE, especially if the rest of clinical picture is consistent with the diagnosis of acute STEMI (Figure 4.1).

A "NORMAL VARIANT" PATTERN OF NISTE

A "normal variant" STE is defined as STE mainly in leads V_1-V_3 (Figure 4.2).[5] It is common in young males, mainly African American and Hispanic. In contrast to the NISTE seen in patients with LVH, there are no QRS voltage criteria for LVH present, and there is no concomitant ST depression in the lateral leads. Some investigators do not differentiate between a "normal variant" pattern and "early repolarization" pattern, lumping all together as "early repolarization." Indeed, many patients have both "normal variant" and

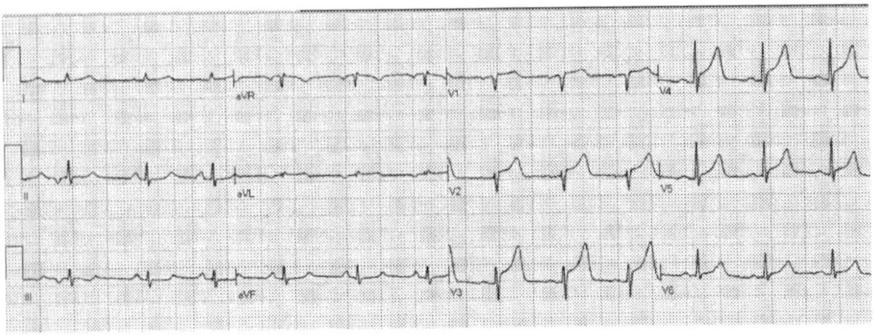

Figure 4.1

Presenting ECG of a 66-year-old man with acute anterior STEMI. ECG shows sinus rhythm and concave ST elevation in leads V_2-V_4. Further, loss of normal R-wave progression in the precordial leads is suggestive of ongoing myocardial necrosis, especially in the absence of criteria for LVH or bundle branch block. Emergent coronary angiography revealed occlusion of his left anterior descending coronary artery, and he underwent PPCI.

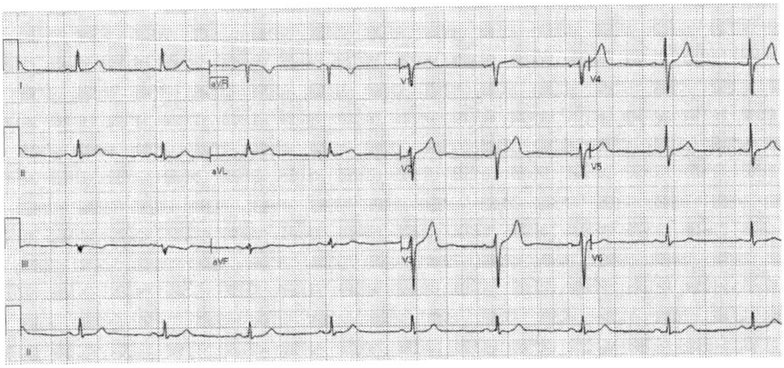

Figure 4.2

A normal variant STE in a young man. There is mild STE with concave pattern in leads V_1-V_4.

"early repolarization" patterns. As mentioned earlier, on the basis of the results of such population studies, the Universal Definition of Myocardial Infarction has narrowed the diagnosis of STEMI as STEs with a J-point of >0.2 mV in men above the age of 40 years and >0.15 mV in women in leads V_2-V_3

and/or >0.1 mV in all other leads,[13] rather than STE at the J-point of >0.1 mV in all other leads as mentioned by the ACCF/AHA guidelines.[1]

EARLY REPOLARIZATION

The typical pattern of early-repolarization NISTE shows STE in the lateral leads (mainly V_5-V_6). It may also involve the inferior leads. There is a characteristic notch at the J-point (Figure 4.3). The ST segment is usually concave, and tall, peaked T waves may be present. Early-repolarization NISTE is commonly seen in young males. In many cases, STE is transient and ameliorates or even disappears with tachycardia and hyperventilation. Thus, dynamic changes in the degree of STE are not always indicative of ischemia.

There is a controversy regarding the underlying pathophysiology of "early repolarization," because it has been demonstrated that this pattern is not associated with early timing of repolarization of the ventricle, suggesting that this term is misleading.[18] Another explanation for the early repolarization pattern may have to do with the regional disparity of transient outward potassium current (I_{to}) channels in the myocardium. I_{to} channels

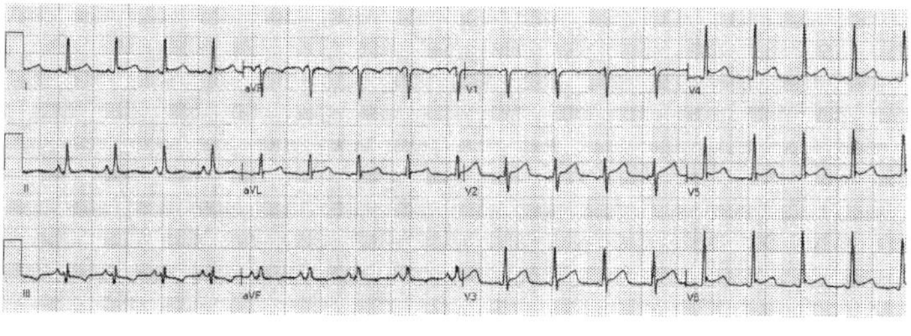

Figure 4.3

An ECG of a young male. ECG shows sinus rhythm with ST elevation and prominent J-point notches in the inferior and precordial leads (V_4-V_6), typical of early repolarization.

are known to be active during phase I of the myocardial action potential, and it is believed that there are more I_{to} channels in the epicardium than in the endocardium. This difference in the relative number of I_{to} channels (and thus K^+ efflux) may lead to a transmural voltage gradient, which manifests as STE or J-point elevation during early repolarization in some individuals. At slow heart rates, a disproportionate increase in K^+ efflux through I_{to} channels in the epicardium may lead to concave STE seen in those with early repolarization.[19] For a long time, early repolarization NISTE was thought to be a benign phenomenon and widely considered to be a normal variant, as this finding is represented in approximately 5% of the population.[20] However, more recently it has been associated with arrhythmic cardiac death, especially if there is >0.2 mV STE.[20-23]

It should be remembered that hypothermia may cause transient prominent J-point notching (Osborne waves)[24] that should not be mistaken for benign early repolarization. Often hypothermia is also associated with bradycardia and tremor. Osborne waves with STE may be seen also in severe hypercalcemia and nervous system disorders. Hypothermia may cause QT prolongation, whereas hypercalcemia is usually associated with short QT interval.[25] Hyperkalemia is a well-known cause of ST-segment elevation, but will also usually present with QRS widening and changes to the PR segment. Another phenomenon that can be confused with J-point notching is the presence of epsilon waves that are seen in arrhythmogenic right ventricular dysplasia (ARVD). However, in ARVD epsilon waves are seen in leads V_1-V_3.[26] ARVD may also be associated with ventricular tachycardia arising from the right ventricular outflow tract (LBBB morphology, superior axis).[27]

ACUTE PERICARDITIS

The classical ECG pattern of acute pericarditis is diffuse STE in all leads, except V_1 and aVR, which instead may show ST

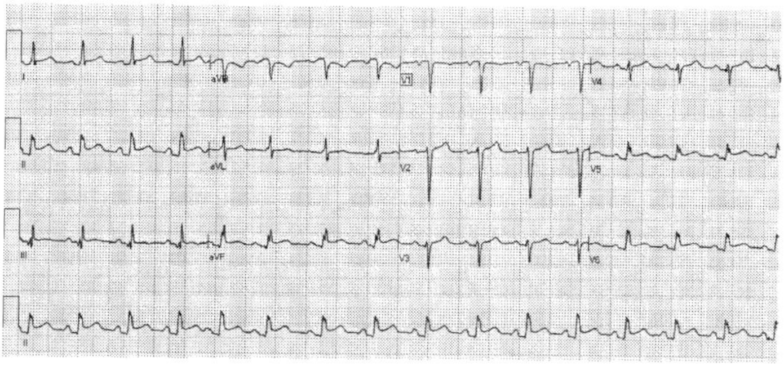

Figure 4.4

An ECG of a patient with acute pericarditis. There is diffuse ST elevation in leads I, II, II, aVF, V_2-V_6 with ST depression in aVR and V_1. Note PR segment depression, suggesting early phase of acute pericarditis.

depression (Figure 4.4). Usually the pattern of STE in pericarditis does not fit a single vascular territory. Depression of the PR interval below the isoelectric line is commonly seen early in the course of pericarditis. However, focal pericarditis following STEMI or cardiac surgery may result in more localized and atypical forms of STE, which may also include ST depression in leads other than aVR and V_1, mimicking myocardial infarction from an isolated coronary artery. Acute (myo-)pericarditis may even be associated with elevated cardiac troponin, perhaps confusing the picture.

STE SECONDARY TO LVH

NISTE secondary to LVH is typically seen in leads V_1-V_3. The cutoffs for STEMI in leads V_2-V_3 do not apply if LVH is present.[13] Usually, there are QRS criteria for LVH and concomitant ST depression in the lateral leads V_5-V_6 (Figure 4.5). In many cases, there is also STE in lead aVR. It is important not to confuse this pattern with the pattern reported to be related to left main related or global ischemia (STE in leads aVR and V_1 with ST depression in the inferior and anterolateral leads).

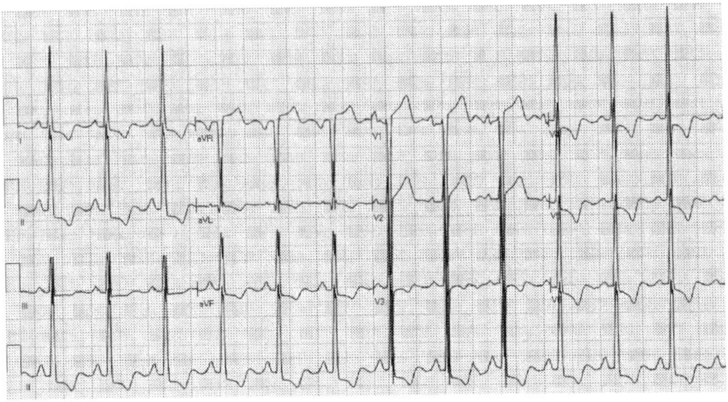

Figure 4.5

An ECG of a patient with severe LVH and repolarization changes. There are criteria for biatrial enlargement. There is marked STE in leads V_1-V_2 and aVR. So-called "strain pattern" is seen on this ECG as marked ST depression in the inferior and lateral leads.

However, LVH may cause atypical patterns of STE (Figure 4.6). Moreover, sometimes patients may have more than one type of NISTE [LVH + early repolarization or LVH + nonspecific intraventricular conduction delay (IVCD)].

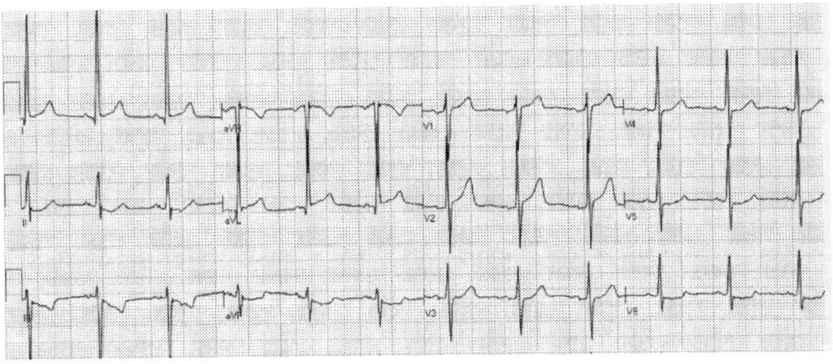

Figure 4.6

An ECG of a 68-year-old male with hypertension. Atypical pattern of STE due to LVH. There is STE instead of the typical ST depression in leads I and aVL. There is mild STE in leads V_1-V_2, but not in lead V_3. In addition, there is ST depression with positive terminal T waves in the inferior leads and leads V_5-V_6.

STE SECONDARY TO IVCD AND/OR ALTERED DEPOLARIZATION

LBBB is commonly associated with marked ST changes (Figure 4.7). ST deviation is usually discordant to the direction of the major deflection of the QRS complex. Acute myocardial infarction (AMI), on the other hand, is more likely to be with primary ST-T wave abnormalities where ST-T wave deviation is concordant to the QRS complex. Because patients with LBBB usually have negative QRS deflections in leads V_1-V_3, they usually display prominent STE in those leads. Sgarbossa et al.[28,29] published criteria on how to differentiate NISTE from STEMI in patients with LBBB. The 3 ECG criteria for STEMI in these patients are: (1) STE >0.1 mV that is concordant with the QRS complex; (2) ST depression >0.1 mV in lead V_1, V_2, or V_3; and (3) STE >0.5 mV that was discordant with the QRS complex. These criteria were validated by Al-Faleh et al.[30] However, these criteria cannot often be relied upon, as they have very low sensitivity (0%–16%) for identifying AMI in patients with LBBB.[31,32] It should be remembered that the magnitude of ST deviation in patients with LBBB is highly

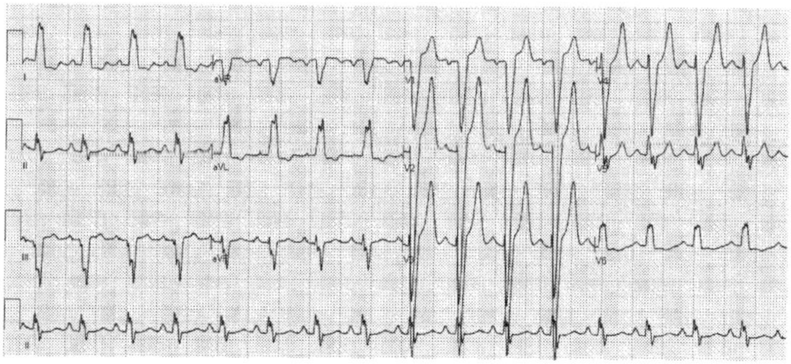

Figure 4.7

A patient with sinus rhythm and LBBB. There is marked STE in the leads with negative QRS configuration (V_1-V_4). In contrast, ST depression is seen in leads with predominantly positive QRS deflection (I, aVL, V_6).

dependent on the degree of aberrancy and may change when QRS duration or heart rate varies. Also, the degree of ST deviation may differ between repeated tracings owing to variability in the placement of the electrodes on the chest wall; this is especially pronounced in the anterolateral precordial leads in patients with left axis deviation.

Similar to LBBB, patients with nonspecific IVCD may also have NISTE secondary to repolarization changes (Figure 4.8). The pattern of ST deviation in these patients varies and accurate diagnosis can only be made by comparing the presenting ECG to previous tracings or by following dynamic changes in subsequent tracings.

Right bundle branch block (RBBB) usually does not interfere with interpretation of ST deviation. However, patients with RBBB may display ST depression in the precordial leads V_1-V_3 that may increase with tachycardia. This pattern of ST depression should not be confused with true inferolateral (posterior) STEMI. Actually, there are no criteria stating how to diagnose "true" inferolateral (posterior) STEMI equivalent in patients with RBBB. Similar to LBBB, concordant ST segment shifts with "flipping" of the ST segment and T waves in

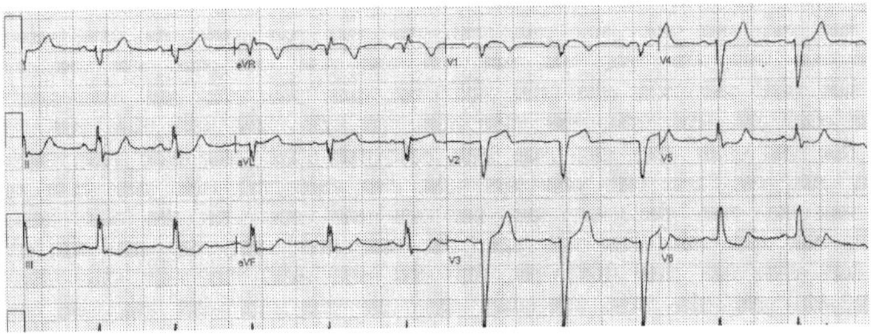

Figure 4.8

An ECG of an 83-year-old man with heart failure and coronary artery disease. At the time of ECG recording, the patient was stable and asymptomatic. There is sinus rhythm with nonspecific IVCD. There is minimal STE in lead aVL and significant STE in leads V_1-V_3. There is also ST depression in the inferior leads and V_5-V_6.

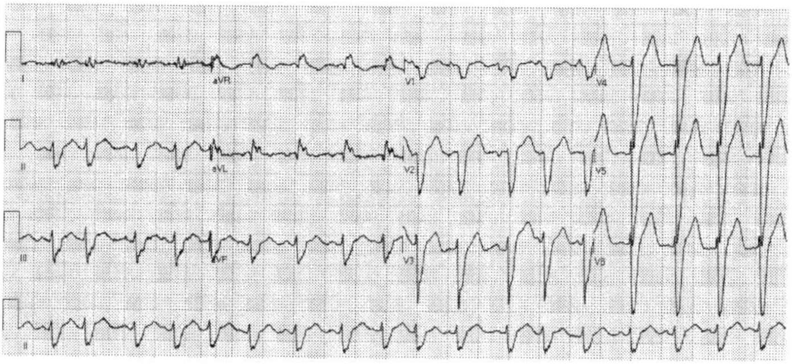

Figure 4.9

An ambulatory ECG of a patient with sinus rhythm and RBBB + left anterior fascicular block. There is minimal ST elevation in the inferior leads and marked STE in leads V_2-V_6.

the same direction as the major QRS deflection is highly suspicious of transmural ischemia. However, occasionally NISTE can be seen in patients with RBBB, especially those with cardiomyopathies (Figure 4.9).

Another scenario more commonly encountered today is patients with electronic ventricular pacing. These patients commonly have secondary ST-T changes that may be dynamic, especially in patients with biventricular pacing. At present, no published criteria exist to distinguish this form of NISTE from STEMI.

Wolff-Parkinson-White (WPW) pattern may also cause NISTE owing to repolarization abnormalities that are secondary to the depolarization changes (Figure 4.10). The degree of ST deviation is highly dependent on the degree of activation via the accessory pathway.

THE BRUGADA PATTERN

The Brugada pattern of NISTE shows a RBBB pattern with STE in the anterior leads (Figure 4.11).[33,34] The Brugada pattern is

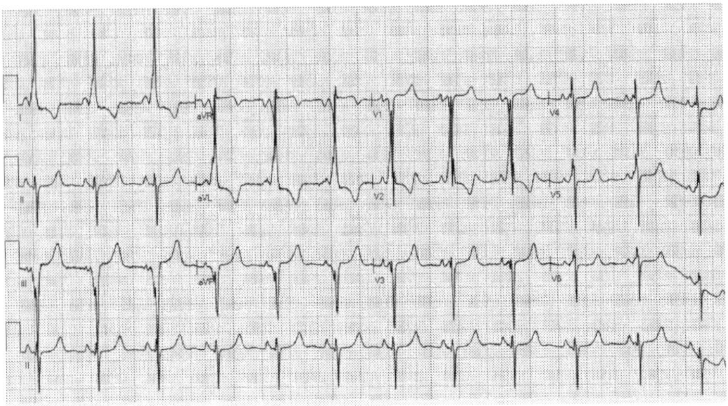

Figure 4.10

An ECG of a patient with WPW and obvious anterograde manifest conduction through an accessory pathway. Huge negative delta waves are seen in the inferior leads, mimicking Q waves. Mild ST elevation with tall positive T waves is seen in the inferior leads. Positive delta waves in leads I and aVL, superior axis, and early precordial delta wave transition (V_1-V_2) are suggestive of the presence of a right paraseptal accessory pathway.

associated with a high risk for ventricular tachyarrhythmia and sudden cardiac death. Type 1 Brugada is characterized by a coved STE > 0.2 mV followed by a negative T wave in more than one of the right precordial leads (V_1-V_3) in the presence

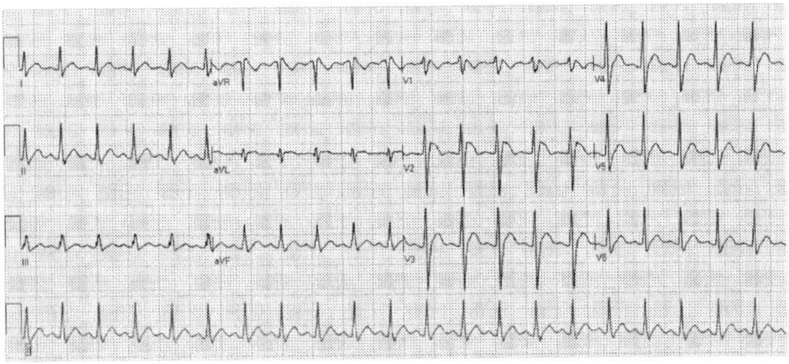

Figure 4.11

A typical ECG of a patient with a type 1 Brugada pattern. There is RSR' pattern with ST elevation and negative T waves in leads V_1-V_2.

or absence of a sodium channel blocker and in conjunction with documented clinical risk factors such as ventricular fibrillation, polymorphic ventricular tachycardia, a family history of sudden cardiac death at age < 45 years, similar ECG pattern in relatives, inducibility of ventricular tachycardia with programmed electrical stimulation, syncope, or nocturnal agonal respiration.[35] Type 2 Brugada has STE with a saddleback pattern with initial STE of > 0.2 mV that decreases in the mid portion and distal portion with a positive or biphasic T wave. Type 3 Brugada pattern has STE with either a saddleback or coved pattern of STE < 0.1 mV. Type 2 and 3 patterns are not diagnostic of the Brugada syndrome, as they can also be benign patterns in the general population. The ECG changes of the Brugada pattern are dynamic and may change over time, with different types of STE seen on different days.[34]

TAKOTSUBO SYNDROME (APICAL BALLOONING SYNDROME)

Apical ballooning syndrome (also called "Takotsubo") is more common in postmenopausal women and classically occurs following acute emotional or physiologic stress. Presentation is often confused with STEMI, because patients may complain of chest pain or an anginal equivalent such as shortness of breath and their ECG may show STE (81.6% of the patients, mainly in the precordial leads), T-wave abnormalities (64.3%), and Q waves (31.8%). Mild elevation of cardiac markers has been reported in 86.2% of the patients.[36] In many cases, the initial presentation is indistinguishable from anterior STEMI, although evaluation of left ventricular function by echocardiogram may show apical distribution of regional wall motion abnormalities that is not typical of anterior STEMI. However, the ECG of classical Takotsubo is indistinguishable from STEMI caused by a distal occlusion of an apex-wrapping LAD (STE in the anterior and inferior leads). It has recently been suggested that at later ECG stages, when T waves become negative in

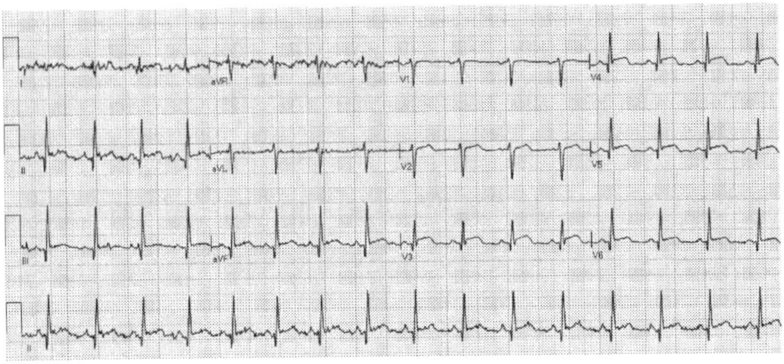

Figure 4.12

An ECG of a 73-year-old female with Takotsubo syndrome. Coronary angiography did not show significant coronary narrowing. ECG shows narrow Q waves in the inferior leads, mild ST elevation in the inferior leads + leads V_3-V_6.

the precordial leads, patients with Takotsubo more often have positive T-waves in lead aVR and lack T-wave inversion in lead V_1.[37] Patients with Takotsubo may also have more extensive ST-segment deviation in lead aVR and less ST-segment deviation in lead V_1 compared with those with acute, anterior myocardial infarction.[38] Acute cerebral infarction (particularly with subarachnoid hemorrhage)[39,40] and pheochromocytoma[41,42] can present with similar ECG and echocardiographic findings as Takotsubo cardiomyopathy. Figure 4.12 is an example of a patient with Takotsubo syndrome.

LEFT VENTRICULAR ANEURYSM

Left ventricular aneurysm may cause persistent STE following a previous myocardial infarction that, at times, may be indistinguishable from acute STEMI (Figure 4.13). Diagnosis is especially difficult when previous ECG tracings are unavailable. Usually, pathologic Q waves are present in the same leads as those with STE when LV aneurysm is present. The

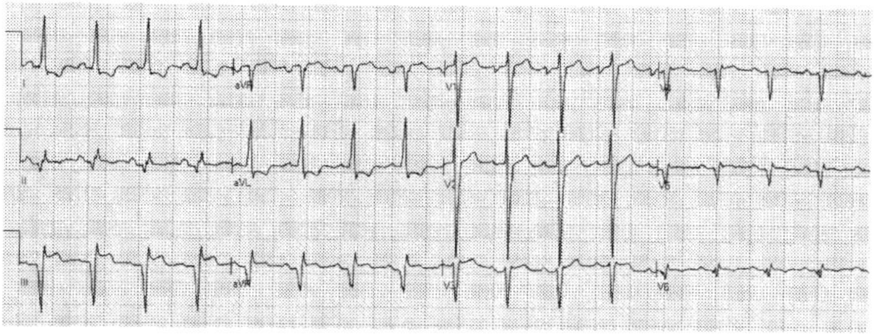

Figure 4.13

An ECG of a 50-year-old woman with systemic lupus erythematosus and coronary artery disease. She had a myocardial infarction few years earlier. ECG shows Q waves in the inferior leads and V_4-V_6, indicating old infarction. There are tall R waves in leads V_1-V_2, indicating old inferolateral (posterior) infarction. In addition, there is ST elevation in the inferolateral leads. Patient denied chest pain. Her cardiac markers were negative. Transthoracic echocardiogram revealed an inferior aneurysm of the left ventricle proving that ST elevations in the inferolateral leads were in fact chronic.

magnitude of STE may be dependent on the heart rate and, in contrast to early repolarization, increases with fast heart rates.

SPONTANEOUSLY REPERFUSED STEMI

The current ACCF/AHA guidelines for STEMI recommend that patients with symptoms suggestive of myocardial ischemia but without evidence of STE in two or more adjacent ECG leads should be managed conservatively rather than given immediate reperfusion therapy,[1] because those with non-ST elevation acute coronary syndrome (NSTE-ACS) do not usually have totally occlusive thrombosis of the culprit epicardial vessel during coronary angiography and fail to achieve benefit with emergent (< 12 hours) primary reperfusion. However, the guidelines do not mention the entity of spontaneously reperfused STEMI (i.e., when a totally occlusive thrombus recannulates allowing some degree of flow to the distal segments of the culprit vessel before primary reperfusion can be performed), and they do not mention ongoing symptoms as a prerequisite for immediate reperfusion therapy if presented within 12 hours of onset of symptoms. A significant number of patients present with complete or at least partial resolution of symptoms on arrival to the hospital, especially if chewable aspirin was given earlier. Their ECG may show complete or partial STE resolution with terminal T-wave inversion compared with a prehospital ECG (if performed). While these patients are at risk of reocclusion, it is unknown at this time whether this subset of patients with AMI have the same benefit with emergent primary reperfusion therapy as other patients with STEMI who have ongoing symptoms and whose ECG shows ST elevation with upright T waves. Randomized clinical trials have not addressed the role of reperfusion therapy (thrombolysis or PPCI) in this subset of patients.

CONCLUSION

The benefits of reperfusion therapy are time dependent in those with true, acute STEMI, and rapid ECG interpretation is vital in strategies aimed to reduce door-to-balloon times.[43] The ACCF/AHA STEMI guidelines state that the physician in the Emergency Department should make a diagnosis of STEMI within 10 minutes of performing the initial ECG.[1,10] Since the establishment of nationalized quality-of-care measures,[44] institutional door-to-balloon times have been improving in the United States. Some of the technology advances that make a system approach for early ECG interpretation available have been discussed in the previous chapter. Controversy remains regarding which personnel and what training are needed to maximize the diagnostic advantage of the ECG obtained in the field. One such strategy is wireless prehospital transmission of ECGs by emergency medical services (EMS) to experienced on-call cardiologists.[45] This strategy has been shown to reduce door-to-balloon time[46] and door-to-needle time.[47] However, in this setting, the ECG interpretation must be made without the benefit of personally taking a patient history, or being able to perform a physical examination or review the patients' previous ECGs. Although such strategy may improve the sensitivity of detecting STE, it is unclear how it will affect specificity and false activation of the catheterization laboratory. One important advance would be new technology that would allow documentation of the clinical conditions while the ECG was recorded (pain, symptom-free, etc.) into the digital ECG machine databases.

In conclusion, the majority of patients with STEMI present with classical ECG patterns of STE. With a combination of history taking, physical examination, and ECG reading, a diagnosis can usually be made. Nevertheless, there are many cases with atypical presentation and ECGs that may actually represent NISTE. Several patterns of NISTE are easy to diagnose (early repolarization, normal pattern, changes secondary to LVH, etc.). However, patients with NISTE may concurrently present with STEMI, non-STEMI, and so on, making the differentiation complex. Moreover, even when previous ECGs are available, the magnitude of NISTE may have dramatically changed over time depending on the degree of depolarization changes and heart rate. In many cases, a definite diagnosis might not be possible according to clinical judgment and ECG alone, and other modalities, such as echocardiography, may be needed to make the right diagnosis.

REFERENCES

1. O'Gara PT, Kushner FG, Ascheim DD, et al. 2013 ACCF/AHA guideline for the management of ST-elevation myocardial infarction: a report of the American College of Cardiology Foundation/American Heart Association task force on practice guidelines. *J Am Coll Cardiol*. 2013;61:e78–e140.

2. Task Force on the management of ST-segment elevation acute myocardial infarction of the European Society of Cardiology (ESC), Steg PG, James SK, Atar D, et al. ESC Guidelines for the management of acute myocardial infarction in patients presenting with ST-segment elevation. *Eur Heart J.* 2012;33:2569–2619.
3. Brady WJ, Perron AD, Martin ML, et al. Cause of ST segment abnormality in ED chest pain patients. *Am J Emerg Med.* 2001;19:25–28.
4. Otto LA, Aufderheide TP. Evaluation of ST segment elevation criteria for the prehospital electrocardiographic diagnosis fo acute myocardial infarction. *Ann Emerg Med.* 1994;23:17–24.
5. Wang K, Asinger RW, Marriott HJ. ST-segment elevation in conditions other than acute myocardial infarction. *N Engl J Med.* 2003;349:2128–2135.
6. Birnbaum Y. The burden of nonischemic ST-segment elevation. *J Electrocardiol.* 2007;40:6–9.
7. Canto JG, Shlipak MG, Rogers WJ, et al. Prevalence, clinical characteristics, and mortality among patients with myocardial infarction presenting without chest pain. *JAMA.* 2000;283:3223–3229.
8. Deedwania PC, Carbajal EV. Silent myocardial ischemia. A clinical perspective. *Arch Intern Med.* 1991;151:2373–2382.
9. Kyker KA, Limacher MC. Gender differences in the presentation and symptoms of coronary artery disease. *Curr Womens Health Rep.* 2002;2:115–119.
10. Zimetbaum PJ, Josephson ME. Use of the electrocardiogram in acute myocardial infarction. *N Engl J Med.* 2003;348:933–940.
11. Larson DM, Menssen KM, Sharkey SW, et al. “False-positive” cardiac catheterization laboratory activation among patients with suspected ST-segment elevation myocardial infarction. *JAMA.* 2007;298:2754–2760.
12. Sejersten M, Sillesen M, Hansen PR, et al. Effect on treatment delay of prehospital teletransmission of 12-lead electrocardiogram to a cardiologist for immediate triage and direct referral of patients with ST-segment elevation acute myocardial infarction to primary percutaneous coronary intervention. *Am J Cardiol.* 2008;101:941–946.
13. Tran V, Huang HD, Diez JG, et al. Differentiating ST-elevation myocardial infarction from non-ischemic ST-elevation in patients with chest pain. *Am J Cardiol.* 2011;108(8):1096–1101.
14. Hiss RG, Lamb LE, Allen MF. Electrocardiographic findings in 67,375 asymptomatic subjects. X. Normal values. *Am J Cardiol.* 1960;6:200–231.
15. Surawicz B, Parikh SR. Prevalence of male and female patterns of early ventricular repolarization in the normal ECG of males and females from childhood to old age. *J Am Coll Cardiol.* 2002;40:1870–1876.

16. Thygesen K, Alpert JS, Jaffe AS, et al. Third universal definition of myocardial infarction. *Circulation.* 2012;126:2020–2035.
17. Smith SW. Upwardly concave ST segment morphology is common in acute left anterior descending coronary occlusion. *J Emerg Med.* 2006;31:69–77.
18. Mirvis DM. Evaluation of normal variations in S-T segment patterns by body surface isopotential mapping: S-T segment elevation in absence of heart disease. *Am J Cardiol.* 1982;50:122–128.
19. Zimetbaum PJ, Josephson ME. *Practical Clinical Electrophysiology.* Philadelphia, PA: Lippincott Williams and Wilkins; 2009.
20. Klatsky AL, Oehm R, Cooper RA, et al. The early repolarization normal variant electrocardiogram: Correlates and consequences. *Am J Med.* 2003;115:171–177.
21. Tikkanen JT, Anttonen O, Junttila MJ, et al. Long-term outcome associated with early repolarization on electrocardiography. *N Engl J Med.* 2009;361:2529–2537.
22. Haissaguerre M, Derval N, Sacher F, et al. Sudden cardiac arrest associated with early repolarization. *N Engl J Med.* 2008;358:2016–2023.
23. Nam GB, Kim YH, Antzelevitch C. Augmentation of J waves and electrical storms in patients with early repolarization. *N Engl J Med.* 2008;358:2078–2079.
24. Spodick DH. Hypothermia with J (Osborne) waves. *Am Heart Hosp J.* 2006;4:156.
25. Nishi SP, Barbagelata NA, Atar S, et al. Hypercalcemia-induced ST-segment elevation mimicking acute myocardial infarction. *J Electrocardiol.* 2006;39:298–300.
26. Nasir K, Bomma C, Tandri H, et al. Electrocardiographic features of arrhythmogenic right ventricular dysplasia/cardiomyopathy according to disease severity: A need to broaden diagnostic criteria. *Circulation.* 2004;110:1527–1534.
27. Cox MG, van der Smagt JJ, Noorman M, et al. Arrhythmogenic right ventricular dysplasia/cardiomyopathy diagnostic task force criteria: Impact of new task force criteria. *Circ Arrhythm Electrophysiol.* 2010;3(2):126–133.
28. Sgarbossa EB. Value of the ECG in suspected acute myocardial infarction with left bundle branch block. *J Electrocardiol.* 2000;33(suppl):87–92.
29. Sgarbossa EB, Pinski SL, Barbagelata A, et al. Electrocardiographic diagnosis of evolving acute myocardial infarction in the presence of left bundle-branch block. GUSTO-1 (Global Utilization of Streptokinase and Tissue Plasminogen Activator for Occluded Coronary Arteries) Investigators. *N Engl J Med.* 1996;334:481–487.
30. Al-Faleh H, Fu Y, Wagner G, et al. Unraveling the spectrum of left bundle branch block in acute myocardial infarction: Insights from

the Assessment of the Safety and Efficacy of a New Thrombolytic (ASSENT 2 and 3) trials. *Am Heart J.* 2006;151:10–15.

31. Li SF, Walden PL, Marcilla O, et al. Electrocardiographic diagnosis of myocardial infarction in patients with left bundle branch block. *Ann Emerg Med.* 2000;36:561–565.
32. Gula LJ, Dick A, Massel D. Diagnosing acute myocardial infarction in the setting of left bundle branch block: prevalence and observer variability from a large community study. *Coron Artery Dis.* 2003;14:387–393.
33. Antzelevitch C, Nof E. Brugada syndrome: Recent advances and controversies. *Curr Cardiol Rep.* 2008;10:376–383.
34. Brugada P, Brugada R, Brugada J. The Brugada syndrome. *Curr Cardiol Rep.* 2000;2:507–514.
35. Antzelevitch C, Brugada P, Borggrefe M, et al. Brugada syndrome: Report of the second consensus conference: endorsed by the Heart Rhythm Society and the European Heart Rhythm Association. *Circulation.* 2005;111:659–670.
36. Gianni M, Dentali F, Grandi AM, et al. Apical ballooning syndrome or takotsubo cardiomyopathy: A systematic review. *Eur Heart J.* 2006;27:1523–1529.
37. Kosuge M, Kimura K, Morita S, et al. Abstract 3267: Positive T wave in lead aVR and no negative T wave in lead V1 distinguishes Takotsubo cardiomyopathy from recanalized anterior acute myocardial infarction. *Circulation.* 2009;120:S775-c.
38. Kosuge M, Ebina T, Hibi K, et al. Simple and accurate electrocardiographic criteria to differentiate takotsubo cardiomyopathy from anterior acute myocardial infarction. *J Am Coll Cardiol.* 2010;55:2514–2516.
39. Rahimi AR, Katayama M, Mills J. Cerebral hemorrhage: Precipitating event for a takotsubo-like cardiomyopathy? *Clin Cardiol.* 2008;31:275–280.
40. Santana-Cabrera L, Escot CR, Medina Gil JM, et al. Takotsubo cardiomyopathy associated with acute subarachnoid hemorrhage. *J Emerg Med.* 2010; 42:586–587.
41. Lassnig E, Weber T, Auer J, et al. Pheochromocytoma crisis presenting with shock and takotsubo-like cardiomyopathy. *Int J Cardiol.* 2009;134:e138–e140.
42. Takizawa M, Kobayakawa N, Uozumi H, et al. A case of transient left ventricular ballooning with pheochromocytoma, supporting pathogenetic role of catecholamines in stress-induced cardiomyopathy or takotsubo cardiomyopathy. *Int J Cardiol.* 2007;114:e15–e17.
43. Bradley EH, Herrin J, Wang Y, et al. Strategies for reducing the door-to-balloon time in acute myocardial infarction. *N Engl J Med.* 2006;355:2308–2320.

44. Jacobs AK, Antman EM, Faxon DP, Gregory T, Solis P. Development of systems of care for ST-elevation myocardial infarction patients: Executive summary. *Circulation*. 2007;116:217–230.

45. Garvey JL, MacLeod BA, Sopko G, et al. Pre-hospital 12-lead electrocardiography programs: a call for implementation by emergency medical services systems providing advanced life support--National Heart Attack Alert Program (NHAAP) Coordinating Committee; National Heart, Lung, and Blood Institute (NHLBI); National Institutes of Health. *J Am Coll Cardiol*. 2006;47:485–491.

46. Dhruva VN, Abdelhadi SI, Anis A, et al. ST-Segment Analysis Using Wireless Technology in Acute Myocardial Infarction (STAT-MI) trial. *J Am Coll Cardiol*. 2007;50:509–513.

47. Terkelsen CJ, Norgaard BL, Lassen JF, et al. Telemedicine used for remote prehospital diagnosing in patients suspected of acute myocardial infarction. *J Intern Med*. 2002;252:412–420.

CHAPTER 5

Triage Models for ST-Elevation Myocardial Infarction Systems of Prehospital Care and the Challenge of Inappropriate Cardiac Catheterization Laboratory Activation

David A. Hildebrandt, RN, NREMTP, David M. Larson, MD, and Timothy D. Henry, MD

INTRODUCTION

Early heart attack symptom recognition with rapid diagnosis and timely access to reperfusion is essential in patients suffering from acute ST-elevation myocardial infarction (STEMI) and is associated with decreased morbidity and mortality.[1,2] The immediate goal in the STEMI patient is to restore coronary flow and myocardial tissue perfusion as quickly as possible. Primary percutaneous coronary intervention (PPCI) is the preferred reperfusion strategy when it can be accomplished within 90 minutes of patient arrival at the hospital.[3,4] The time

Prehospital Management of Acute STEMI: Practical Approaches and International Strategies for Early Intervention © 2015 Joseph S. Alpert, Lynne T. Braun, Barbara J. Fletcher, Gerald Fletcher, Editors-in-Chief, Cardiotext Publishing, ISBN: 978-1-935395-66-9

after arrival at the hospital until the time of device deployment is defined as the door-to-balloon time (D2B). Fibrinolysis is used as a secondary reperfusion strategy in the STEMI patient in which PPCI is not possible within 90 minutes of arrival.[3] The 2013 American College of Cardiology Foundation (ACCF)/ American Heart Association (AHA) STEMI guidelines recommend PPCI when first medical contact-to-balloon time is <90 minutes (first medical contact defined as the time of contact with emergency medical services [EMS] or time of arrival to the emergency department [ED]) in patients who present to a PCI hospital and <120 minutes in those patients who present to a non-PCI-capable hospital and require transfer.[3]

The emphasis on reducing door-to-reperfusion times under the premise that "time is muscle" is supported by multiple studies that have shown a decrease in time to treatment improves mortality.[3,5] Initiatives such as the ACC's D2B Alliance and the AHA's Mission: Lifeline were created to implement strategies that reduce D2B time and foster the development of STEMI systems of care, which would increase the number of patients who have timely access to PPCI in the United States.[1,6-11]

Rapid triage and identification of the STEMI patient with subsequent activation of the "STEMI system" by a wide range of healthcare providers, including the emergency medical technician (EMT) basic provider, EMT paramedic, nurse, physician's assistant, and/or ED physician, is an important strategy used to reduce D2B time. STEMI identification in the prehospital setting by EMS or at the PCI- or non-PCI-capable hospital requires providers experienced in 12-lead ECG interpretation, as reviewed in Chapter 4. One of the potential downfalls of this strategy is the inherit risk of the "false positive" or "inappropriate cardiac catheterization laboratory (CCL) activation." This chapter addresses this concern in detail. We will look at current and ideal prehospital triage models in STEMI systems with a focus on the challenging issue of "false positive" or "inappropriate CCL activation" and include steps to reduce the rate of these "false alarms," which can be a drain on financial and emotional resources.

SYSTEMS OF CARE APPROACH: IDEAL FEATURES

In an ideal STEMI system, patients experiencing acute coronary syndrome symptoms would quickly seek medical help and access the 911 system. EMS arrival would place priority on rapid acquisition of an ECG and quick triage of the patient. All EMS units would have the ability to perform an ECG. Although continued effort is being made to increase the number of EMS units with the ability to acquire prehospital ECG, many still do not, especially in rural areas. Lack of prehospital ECG capability is frequently due to lack of funds to purchase equipment and/or funds to properly train EMS providers. In some instances, charitable foundations have provided funds to support community-based STEMI systems. For example, in 2010, the Helmsley Charitable Trust awarded the AHA an $8.4 million grant to build a STEMI system for South Dakota. As part of the grant, every EMS unit in the state received a monitor capable of ECG acquisition and transmission. Expansion of this same project is underway in both North Dakota and rural parts of Minnesota.[12]

In an urban setting, paramedics would quickly obtain the ECG and either transmit the ECG to the receiving PCI-capable hospital (which would then confirm STEMI and activate the STEMI process), or interpret the ECG themselves and activate the CCL from the field, if STEMI was identified. EMS would bypass any non-PCI-capable hospital in the urban setting and transport the patient directly to a PCI-capable hospital. On arrival to the PCI hospital, the patient would bypass the ED and immediately be taken to the CCL for immediate angiography and reperfusion.

In the rural setting (which often utilizes basic life-support EMS units), where STEMI patients must be transferred from a non-PCI-capable hospital to a PCI-capable hospital, the ECG would be transmitted by EMS to both the non-PCI-capable and PCI-capable hospital (in rural areas served by paramedics, the ECG should be acquired, interpreted by the paramedics, and the STEMI system activated as in an urban region). Once STEMI is confirmed, interfacility transport (which may include helicopter EMS) is immediately dispatched to transfer the patient to the PCI-capable facility. One call is made from the non-PCI-capable hospital to the PCI-capable hospital and the STEMI team is activated. On arrival to the non-PCI hospital, simplified, standard protocols are implemented to rapidly prepare the patient for transport, administer adjunctive medications, and perform essential lab studies with a door-in-door-out goal of < 30 minutes. Then, EMS transports the STEMI patient to the PCI-capable hospital and takes the patient directly to the CCL for PPCI.

ROLE OF EMS

EMS plays an essential role in the STEMI system, and EMS acquisition of the prehospital ECG reduces time to reperfusion when prehospital STEMI diagnosis and activation of the CCL occur. A decrease in D2B times of 15 to 20 minutes has been reported as a result of prehospital ECG acquisition, which can be even more substantial when the CCL team is activated from the prehospital setting.[13]

Most urban EMS systems have the ability to acquire a prehospital ECG and increasingly paramedics are allowed to either activate the CCL team after interpretation of the ECG, or transmit the ECG to the receiving hospital for a physician to confirm before activating the CCL. In Minneapolis/St. Paul, MN, paramedics (< 500 total) are allowed to activate the CCL team without physician interpretation if the patient has an ECG computer algorithm that reports STEMI, and the paramedic over-read agrees with the interpretation in a patient with ischemic symptoms (chest pain, dyspnea, nausea).[12] Patients with left bundle branch block (LBBB) are evaluated in the ED. Standardized protocols may also recommend to exclude patients with arrhythmias or borderline ST-elevation from CCL activation but with an alert to the ED physician. ECG education and retraining may be challenging in certain regions, and ECG transmission may be the best option.

The success of prehospital regional STEMI systems was recently demonstrated in a pooled analysis of 10 metropolitan, independent regional STEMI-receiving center networks. In this analysis, 2712 patients with a prehospital diagnosis of STEMI after ECG acquisition had emergent PPCI performed in 2053 (76%) of the cases, and 86% of those cases had a D2B time of <90 minutes. However, 24% of the patients did not receive PPCI, and the reasons were not clear. The prehospital ECG acquisition time-to-balloon was <90 minutes in 68% of the cases, illustrating the importance of this strategy.[14] An extension of this strategy to reduce D2B time in the EMS activated CCL for STEMI is to allow the patient to go directly to the CCL from the field by bypassing the ED. In Boston, MA, for example, paramedics bypass the ED for triage when they have a "definite" STEMI, and stop in the ED for triage when they have a "probable" STEMI.[15]

NON-PCI HOSPITALS WITHIN STEMI SYSTEMS

Non-PCI-capable hospitals play an important role in triage of STEMI patients, and processes can be implemented in a STEMI system to reduce D2B time for the transferred patient. All hospitals should have standard triage protocols in place to acquire an ECG within 10 minutes of arrival for any patient that presents with ischemic symptoms. In the non-PCI-capable facility, protocols need to be in place for rapid transfer of the STEMI patient to a PCI-capable facility. PCI-capable facilities should work closely with all associated non-PCI hospitals in the STEMI system to provide a simplified, streamlined process to transport the STEMI patient to the PCI-capable facility on the basis of available local and regional resources, which consider weather, EMS ground-versus-air availability, and traffic patterns. Non-PCI-capable hospitals should notify the PCI-capable hospital with one phone call to activate the CCL at the PCI-capable hospital.

An example is the "Level 1" regional STEMI system at the Minneapolis Heart Institute at Abbott Northwestern Hospital (MHI/ANW), designed in 2002 to provide rapid access to PPCI using a standardized protocol and integrated transfer system for STEMI patients from rural and community hospitals in Minnesota and Wisconsin up to 210 miles from the PCI center.[8,9] Standardized protocols with a few key differences are in place for the PCI center, for zone 1 hospitals (up to 60 miles from the PCI center) and for zone 2 hospitals (61–210 miles from the PCI center (Figure 5.1). The key differences in protocols include the use of a more rapidly acting antiplatelet agent at the PCI center and the use of a pharmacoinvasive approach with half-dose fibrinolytic for zone 2 patients, where delays of greater than 120 minutes may occur because of long-distance transfers.[16]

Briefly, the MHI/ANW Level 1 protocol is as follows: Patients with ischemic symptoms receive an immediate ECG upon arrival to a referral ED (goal for ECG < 5 minutes). For patients with symptom onset < 24 hours and with ST-elevation or new LBBB, the STEMI system is activated with a single call by referring ED physician to MHI/ANW. Activation of the Level 1 program immediately notifies appropriate departments within MHI/ANW, including the cardiac catheterization team, using a group page. An on-site cardiologist is available 24/7

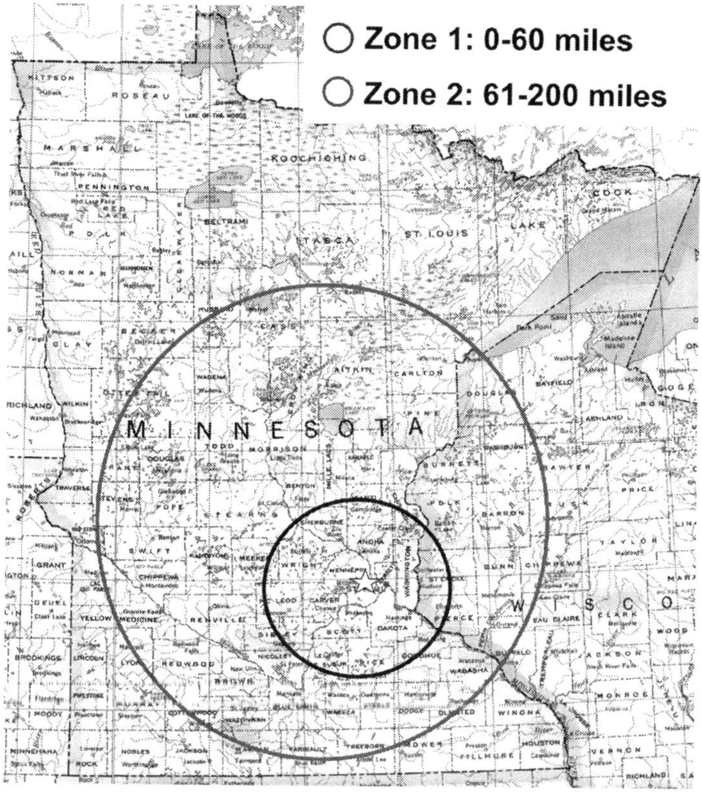

Figure 5.1

Minneapolis Heart Institute "Level 1" Regional STEMI system map with zones.

at MHI/ANW, and in the case of diagnostic uncertainty, the referring physician may fax the ECG to the cardiologist for review before the CCL is activated. Patients receive a standardized protocol of adjunctive medical therapy. Essential laboratory testing is obtained, and results, along with a copy of the patient's ECG, are faxed to the PCI center. On arrival at MHI/ANW, the patient bypasses the ED and is immediately taken to the CCL for PPCI.

"FALSE POSITIVE" AND "INAPPROPRIATE ACTIVATION" OF THE CARDIAC CATH LAB

Empowering EMS or the ED physician to activate the CCL for suspected STEMI according to ECG is clearly one of the most effective strategies to expedite care for the suspected STEMI patient and reduce D2B time. However, "false positive" or "inappropriate activation" of the CCL is a potential challenge and may have negative financial and resource utilization consequences. Excess CCL cancellations may result in stress on hospital staff and may contribute to tension and mistrust between providers in the CCL and those in EMS and the ED.

Part of the problem in developing effective triage systems is the confusing terminology used to describe the 2 main outcomes associated with cath lab activation. Currently in the literature, both the terminology and definitions are confusing: "false positive," "inappropriate activation," "false activation," or "unnecessary activation" of the CCL have all been used to describe the basic situation of cath lab activation without finding a culprit lesion (Table 5.1).

There are 2 major categories of circumstances leading to cath lab activation that for STEMI does not result in PCI of a culprit lesion:

1) ***Inappropriate cath lab activation*** generally refers to situations in which additional professional consultation results in cancelling the cardiac catheterization (or in retrospect, would have). However, the specific criteria reported in the various studies vary widely (see the following).
2) ***False-positive activation*** generally refers to findings on cardiac catheterization that did not reveal a culprit lesion amenable to PCI, but cardiac catheterization was deemed appropriate.

Table 5.1
Previous literature on cardiac catheterization activation laboratory

First author (year)	Total number of patients	Number of patients (%) false positive/ inappropriate activation	Term	Authors' definition of term
Larson et al. (2007)[21]	1335	123/1335 (9.2%)	False-positive CCL activation	No culprit artery and negative biomarkers.
McCabe et al. (2012)[22]	411	146/411 (36%)	False-positive STEMI diagnosis	Lack of culprit lesion by angiography or by assessment of clinical, electrocardiographic, and biomarker data in the absence of angiography.
Swan et al. (2009)[23]	529	136/529 (25.7%) EMS activated	False-positive triage	No significant coronary artery occlusion by PCI or determined by MD to lack need for PCI.
Garvey et al. (2012)[17]	3973	284/1150 (24.7%) EMS activated 197/1547 (12.3%) non-PCI hospital 115/1276 (9%) PCI hospital	Inappropriate CCL activation	CCL activation cancelled because ECG misinterpreted or if patient deemed not to be a candidate for angiography.

(*Continued*)

Table 5.1
(Continued)

First author (year)	Total number of patients	Number of patients (%) false positive/ inappropriate activation	Term	Authors' definition of term
Baran et al. (2010)[19]	209	53/209 (25.3%) EMS activated	Inappropriate CCL activation	CCL activation cancelled after physician assessment of ECG and patient.
Rokos et al. (2010)[18]	646	20% EMS activated	Inappropriate CCL activation	Cardiologist did not perform emergent angiography.
Barnes et al. (2013)[24]	717	204/717 (28%) EMS and ED activated	False CCL activation	Interventional cardiologist cancelled activation after determining patient did not need require emergent transfer from the ED to the CCL.
Mixon et al. (2012)[25]	345	44/345 (12.8%) EMS and ED activations	ECG inappropriate activation	CCL activation inappropriate because ECG did not meet criteria for STEMI for LBB.

Inappropriate Activation

Recently, the statewide STEMI system in North Carolina reported "inappropriate CCL activations" in 284 of 1150 (24.7%) suspected STEMI patients activated by EMS, 12.3% of suspected STEMI patients presenting to a non-PCI hospital and 7.9% of STEMI patients presenting to a PCI-capable hospital.[17] Activation was considered "inappropriate" if the catheterization was cancelled because of ECG reinterpretation (72% of cases), or if the patient was deemed not to be a candidate for catheterization (age >90, active bleeding, known terminal illness, severe comorbidities), which occurred in the other 28% of patients. In another recent report from Los Angeles County, evaluation of the EMS ECG by paramedics resulted in a 20% rate of "inappropriate activation," defined as no emergency angiography.[18] It is uncertain if any of the "inappropriate activation" patients in these 2 trials ultimately went to the CCL, had an MI, or required revascularization. Baran et al.[19] reported a 25% "inappropriate CCL activation" rate by EMS in St. Paul, MN. In this study, 300 advanced cardiac life support EMS personnel were trained on ECG acquisition and prehospital CCL activation with suspected STEMI, and the protocol allowed patients to go directly to the CCL from the field, if the CCL team was ready on patient arrival.

False-Positive Activation

The 12-lead ECG remains the gold standard to rapidly identify candidates for PPCI in suspected STEMI. However, conditions other than myocardial infarction may cause ST-segment elevation.[20] In the setting of ST-elevation and ischemic symptoms, emergent angiography is appropriate and may serve as an excellent diagnostic tool, balancing the risk of false alarm with the consequence of delayed reperfusion.

Even with "appropriate" activation, not all patients with suspected STEMI will have a clear culprit artery on angiography.

Of 1345 consecutive patients undergoing emergent cardiac catheterization for suspected STEMI at the MHI, 187 (14%) had no clear culprit artery, and cardiac biomarkers were negative in 149 (11.2%). The combination of no clear culprit artery with negative cardiac biomarkers was present in 9.2% of patients and was defined as the "false-positive" rate.[21] It is important to note that 34% of patients with no clear culprit artery had elevated cardiac biomarkers and includes patients with Takotsubo syndrome (stress cardiomyopathy), coronary artery spasm, embolus, and myocarditis. The most common causes of no culprit artery and negative biomarkers were LBBB, previous myocardial infarction, pericarditis, early repolarization, and a non-diagnostic ECG (Figure 5.2). In contrast, a

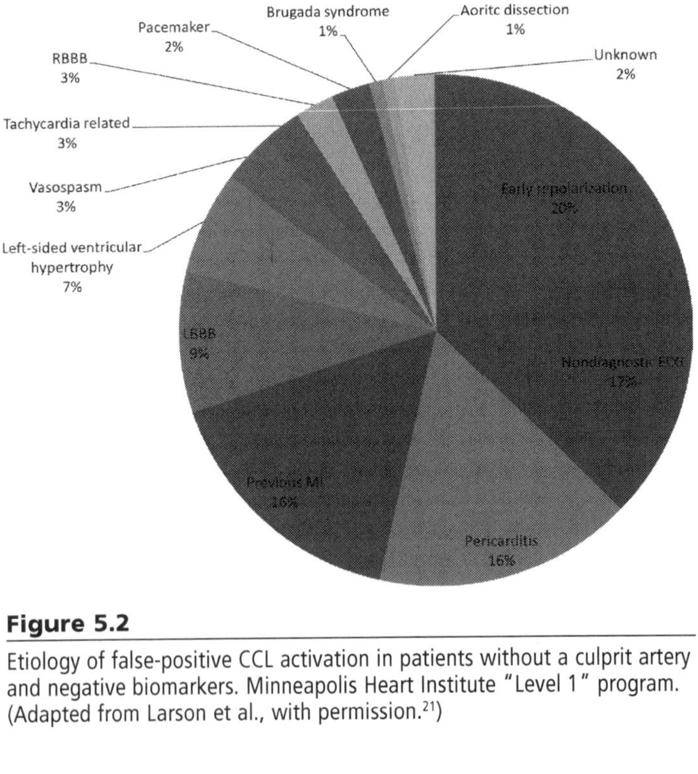

Figure 5.2

Etiology of false-positive CCL activation in patients without a culprit artery and negative biomarkers. Minneapolis Heart Institute "Level 1" program. (Adapted from Larson et al., with permission.[21])

study from 2 STEMI centers in San Francisco reported 36% of consecutive ED patients referred for PPCI had false-positive STEMI cath lab activation.[22] In this study, false positive was defined as lack of a culprit lesion by angiography or by assessment of clinical, electrocardiographic, and biomarker data in the absence of angiography. The term "false-positive STEMI" is misleading. In a patient who presents with ischemic symptoms and ST-elevation on the ECG, immediate cardiac catheterization is quite appropriate, but may not have a clear culprit artery or positive biomarker (false positive), which should not be confused with inappropriate CCL activation due to misreading of the ECG or incomplete evaluation of the patient. The patient with LBBB, previous myocardial infarction, left ventricular aneurysm, or other ST-elevation mimics might be "false positive" but certainly would be "appropriate" for CCL activation. In the MHI/ANW experience, only 1.8% of patients had ECG findings that did not meet criteria for CCL activation.[20]

Standard Definitions Are Needed to Develop Quality Benchmarks

With national efforts to reduce D2B times, concentrated efforts should be deployed to reduce "inappropriate CCL activation." An excellent first step would be to provide standard definitions so that quality benchmarks can be developed. CCL activations should be deemed as either appropriate or inappropriate. Rokos et al.[18] suggests the use of a combined strategy of ECG interpretation and clinical decision to determine the appropriateness of CCL activation. CCL activation cancelled by a physician, ECG misinterpretation, and patients who are not PPCI candidates are all cited as reason to label CCL activation as inappropriate. With retrospective and multidisciplinary review of all index clinical data, Rokos et al. further defines "ideal" appropriate activations (in which angiography and PPCI are performed) and "reasonable" appropriate CCL activations (angiography without PPCI performed when surgical revascularization is indicated; coronary anatomy is not amenable to PCI; alternative STEMI mechanism such as Takotsubo, spasm, or embolism; true STEMI, but patient dies prior to angiography; and angiography with or without PPCI for witnessed, resuscitated, out-of-hospital cardiac arrests from a shockable rhythm) (Table 5.2). In summary, inappropriate CCL activation might best be defined as CCL activation that is cancelled by a physician because of reinterpretation of the ECG or because the patient is not a PPCI candidate.

"False-positive" activation, on the other hand, is based on angiographic findings. In a patient that presents with ischemic symptoms and diagnostic ST-elevation, CCL activation should be considered appropriate, and "false positive" should be defined after angiography based on no clear culprit artery and negative biomarkers. With adoption of this appropriate CCL activation definition, benchmarks can be set and efforts at reducing inappropriate activations can be implemented.

STRATEGIES TO REDUCE INAPPROPRIATE CCL ACTIVATIONS

Multidisciplinary Process Improvement

EMS, ED physicians, and cardiologists meeting frequently to review all EMS activated cases can be very effective for reducing inappropriate CCL activation. In an established prehospital-ECG STEMI-activation program, each agency needs to be aware of their inappropriate CCL activation rate and work toward finding solutions to reduce activations that do not result in the patient going to the CCL. This case review process helps identify common themes which require further education for EMS or ED staff.

Table 5.2
Classification of appropriate versus inappropriate cath lab activation

Appropriate Cath Lab Activation → Ideal
• Angiography and PPCI performed
Appropriate Cath Lab Activation → Reasonable
• Angiography without PPCI performed · Surgical revascularization indicated · Coronary anatomy is not amenable to PPCI intervention (i.e., medical therapy) · No PPCI target-lesion identified but cardiac markers are elevated (STEMI without a true culprit: Takotsubo, embolism, spasm, thrombus resolution) · "Unavoidable angiogram" per index ECG and/or clinical scenario (false positive: LBBB, old MI, LVH, etc.) • Patient dies suddenly before angiography, true STEMI per index ECG • Angiography ± PPCI for ROSC following witnessed OHCA from a shockable rhythm.
Inappropriate Cath Lab Activation → Goal is <5% rate
• No angiography performed (Cath Lab activation cancelled by a physician). · "Emergent caths are at times inappropriately cancelled as well." • Angiography without a PPCI target lesion identified and normal cardiac markers. · "Avoidable angiogram" based upon erroneous ECG interpretation. • Advanced comorbidities: patient is not a PPCI candidate.

Classification based on retrospective and multidisciplinary peer review of all index clinical data. Top Box: ideal scenario. Middle box: events are reasonable. Bottom box: occurrences should be minimized (<5%). ROSC, return of spontaneous circulation; OHCA, out-of-hospital cardiac arrest. (Adapted from Rokos et al.[18] with permission)

Ongoing ECG Education

As ECG misinterpretation appears to be the most common reason for inappropriate activation, EMS personnel should be educated on ECGs that may represent STEMI mimics, such as benign early repolarization, LBBB, pericarditis, left ventricular hypertrophy, paced rhythms, and hyperkalemia, as well as other challenging clinical presentations such as postcardiac arrest and cardiac arrhythmias.[20] Chapter 2 of this book provides detailed information on diagnostic criteria in this setting. Additional training should include evaluating suspected STEMI cases for reciprocal changes, in which appropriate CCL activation is almost certain.[18]

Prehospital Use of the ECG

No matter which EMS strategy is used to reduce D2B time, prehospital use of the ECG is imperative. Collaboration amongst EMS, ED physicians, and cardiologists is essential to continually improve the prehospital STEMI system, reduce D2B times, and increase the percentage of appropriate CCL activations.

Standardized Definitions for "Inappropriate" CCL Activations

As discussed above, standardizing these definitions will make it easier to develop quality benchmarks and process improvement evaluations.

PPCI Internal Hospital Review Process for CCL

PCI-capable hospitals also need to participate in quality and process improvement for their own internal CCL activations and CCL activations from non-PCI capable facilities.

Timely physician feedback and education for ED physicians should focus on eliminating inappropriate activations due to ECG misinterpretations and inappropriate patient selection.

Feedback

Ideally, paramedics should receive immediate feedback when they see the result of the cardiac catheterization, which happens frequently in the MHI Level 1 STEMI program. In addition, as soon as the procedure is complete, the interventional cardiologist calls the ED physicians, and within 24 hours, the attending cardiologist calls the primary care physician. Finally, the PCI hospital STEMI coordinator calls the ED manager and reviews the patient management and results.

CONCLUSION

Significant progress has been made over the last 10 years to reduce time to reperfusion in the suspected STEMI patient. An essential component of a successful STEMI system is prehospital diagnosis, ECG acquisition, and subsequent CCL activation. The interprofessional team involved in this process includes a wide range of healthcare providers such as the basic level EMT, EMT paramedic, nurse, physician's assistant, and/or ED physician as well as the cardiologist. In many geographic areas, especially in the urban setting, prehospital ECG is becoming universal. However, the availability of a prehospital ECG is not uniform throughout the United States and gaps exist, especially in rural areas. As we expand the use of prehospital ECG, we must remain aware of the impact of inappropriate CCL activations, and standard definitions need to be adopted. Ongoing process improvement initiatives should be in place in all successful prehospital STEMI systems.

REFERENCES

1. Krumholz HM, Bradley EH, Nallamothu BK, et al. A campaign to improve the timeliness of primary percutaneous coronary intervention: door to balloon: an alliance for quality. *JACC Cardiovasc Interv.* 2008;1(1):97–104.
2. Lambert L, Brown K, Segal E, et al. Association between timeliness of reperfusion therapy and clinical outcomes in ST-elevation myocardial infarction. *JAMA*. 2010;303(21):2148–2155.
3. O'Gara PT, Kuschner FG, Ascheim DD, et al. 2013 ACCF/AHA guideline for the management of ST-elevation myocardial infarction: executive summary: a report on the American College of Cardiology Foundation/American Heart Association task force on practice guidelines. *Circulation*. 2013;127(4):529–555.
4. Keeley EC, Boura JA, Gaines CL. Primary angioplasty versus intravenous thrombolytic therapy for acute myocardial infarction: a quantitative review of 23 randomised trials. *Lancet*. 2003;361(9351):13–20.
5. Cannon CP, Gibson CM, Lambrew CT, et al. Relationship of symptomatic one-to-balloon time and door-to-balloon time with mortality in patients undergoing anygioplasty for acute myocardial infarction. *JAMA*. 2000;283:2941–2947.
6. Krumholz HM, Herrin J, Miller LE, et al. Improvements in door to balloon time in the United States 2005 to 2010. *Circulation*. 2011;124(9):1038–1045.
7. Jacobs AK, Antman EM, Faxon DP, et al. Development of systems of care for ST-elevation myocardial infarction patients: executive summary. *Circulation*. 2007;116(2):217–230.
8. Henry TD, Unger BT, Sharkey SW, et al. Design of a standardized system for transfer of patients with ST-elevation myocardial infarction for percutaneous coronary intervention. *Am Heart J*. 2005;150(3):373–384.
9. Henry TD, Sharkey SW, Burke MN, et al. A regional system to provide timely access to percutaneous coronary intervention for ST-elevation myocardial infarction. *Circulation*. 2007;116(7):721–728.
10. Bradley EH, Herrin J, Wang Y, et al. Strategies for reducing the door-to-balloon time in acute myocardial infarction. *N Engl J Med*. 2006;255(22):2308–2320.
11. Henry TD, Atikins JM, Cunningham MS, et al. ST-segment elevation myocardial infarction: Recommendations on triage of patients to heart attack centers: is it time for a national policy for the treatment of ST-segment elevation myocardial infarction? *J Am Coll Cardiol*. 2006;47(7):1339–1345.
12. Hildebrandt DA, Larson DM, Henry TD. The critical imperative: Pre-hospital management of the ST-elevation myocardial infarction patient. *Intervent Cardiol Clin*. 2012;1(4):599–608.

13. Ting HH, Krumholz HM, Bradley EH, et al. Implementation and integration of prehospital ECGs into systems of care for acute coronary syndromes: A scientific statement from the American Heart Association Interdisciplinary Council on Quality of Care and Outcomes Research, Emergency Cardiovascular Care Committee, Council on Cardiovascular Nursing, and Council on Clinical Cardiology. *Circulation.* 2008;118(10):1066–1079.
14. Rokos IC, French WJ, Koenig WJ, et al. Integration of pre-hospital electrocardiograms and ST-elevation myocardial infarction receiving center (SRC) networks: impact on door-to-balloon time across 10 independent regions. *JACC Cardiovasc Interv.* 2009;2(4):339–346.
15. Moyer P, Ornato JP, Brady WJ, et al. Development of systems of care for ST-elevation myocardial infarction patients. *Circulation.* 2007;116(2):e43–e48.
16. Larson DM, Duval S, Sharkey SW, et al. Safety and efficacy of a pharmaco-invasive reperfusion strategy in rural ST-elevation myocardial infarction patients with expected delays due to long distance transfers. *Eur Heart J.* 2012;33(10):1232–1240.
17. Garvey JL, Monk L, Granger CB, et al. Rates of cardiac catheterization cancelation for ST-segment elevation myocardial infarction after activation by emergency medical services or emergency physicians: Results from the North Carolina catheterization laboratory activation registry. *Circulation.* 2012;125(2):308–313.
18. Rokos IC, French WJ, Mattu A, et al. Appropriate cardiac cath lab activation: optimizing electrocardiogram interpretation and clinical decision making for acute ST-elevation myocardial infarction. *Am Heart J.* 2010;160(6):995–1003.
19. Baran KW, Kamrowski KA, Westwater JJ, et al. Very rapid treatment of ST-elevation myocardial infarction: utilizing prehospital electrocardiograms to bypass the emergency department. *Circ Cardiovasc Qual Outcomes.* 2010;3(4):431–437.
20. Wang K, Asinger RW, Marriott HJ. ST-segment elevation in conditions other than acute myocardial infarctions. *N Engl J Med.* 2003;349(22):2128–2135.
21. Larson DM, Menseen BA, Sharkey SW, et al. "False positive" cardiac catheterization laboratory activation among patients with suspected ST-segment elevation myocardial infarction. *JAMA.* 2007;298(23):2754–2760.
22. McCabe JM, Armstrong EJ, Kulkarni A, et al. Prevalence and factors associated with false positive ST-segment elevation myocardial diagnoses at primary percutaneous coronary intervention-capable centers. *Arch Intern Med.* 2012;172(11):864–871.
23. Swan PY, Nighswonger B, Boswell GL, Stratton SJ. Factors associated with false-positive emergency medical services triage for percutaneous coronary intervention. *West J Emerg Med.* 2009;10(4):208–212.

24. Barnes GD, Katz A, Desmond JS, et al. False activation of the cardiac catheterization lab for primary PCI. *Am J Manag Care.* 2013;19(8):671–675.
25. Mixon TA, Suhr E, Caldwell G, et al. Retrospective description and analysis of consecutive catheterization laboratory ST-segment elevation myocardial infarction activations with proposal, rationale, and use of a new classification scheme. *Circ Cardiovasc Qual Outcomes.* 2012;5(1):62–69.

CHAPTER 6

Prehospital STEMI Management in the Setting of Out-of-Hospital Cardiac Arrest

Eric Wiel, MD, PhD, and Patrick Goldstein, MD

INTRODUCTION

Patients who have an out-of-hospital cardiac arrest (OHCA) in the course of their ST-segment elevation myocardial infarction (STEMI) represent a special subgroup of prehospital STEMI patients. In spite of much progress in cardiopulmonary resuscitation (CPR), the overall survival rate of OHCA is low, with a long-term survival rate less than 7%.[1] It has been estimated that 90% of OHCAs are due to acute myocardial infarction.[2,3] Only few data on patients with acute STEMI and prehospital CPR are available.[3–6] It has been estimated that 10% to 21% of STEMI patients need defibrillation and CPR.[7–9] A recent registry called Prehospital Myocardial Infarction Registry reported a 10% incidence of STEMI patients who underwent prehospital CPR.[10] Patients with STEMI needing prehospital CPR constitute a subgroup of patients at very high risk for adverse events. The literature reports a high variability in outcomes in such patients due to differences in the definition of the event,

Prehospital Management of Acute STEMI: Practical Approaches and International Strategies for Early Intervention © 2015 Joseph S. Alpert, Lynne T. Braun, Barbara J. Fletcher, Gerald Fletcher, Editors-in-Chief, Cardiotext Publishing, ISBN: 978-1-935395-66-9

its etiology, and the method and timing of coronary reperfusion therapy.

Because primary percutaneous coronary intervention (PPCI) and fibrinolysis have demonstrated good outcomes in the first, "golden" hours of STEMI without CPR, the subgroup of STEMI patients who require CPR (defined as high risk) should benefit logically from such early and aggressive reperfusion treatment.[3-5] However, the role of coronary reperfusion strategies with thrombolysis or PCI in the subgroups of STEMI–OHCA patients remains unclear, although an excellent prognosis of patients with STEMI has been globally reported in the last decade.[11] The literature still gives controversial results, probably owing to limited sample-size studies, retrospective design, or noncomparative analysis between STEMI patients with and without OHCA. Furthermore, the International Liaison Committee on Resuscitation (ILCOR) concludes "there are insufficient data to support or decline the routine use of fibrinolysis in cardiac arrest (CA) from other causes [than pulmonary embolism]."[12]

The main coronary reperfusion strategies available for OHCA patients include thrombolysis, PPCI, and/or adjunct therapies. The aim of this chapter is to review the special characteristics of the STEMI–OHCA population and discuss the state of the art for the therapeutic strategies of OHCA in STEMI patients.

STEMI–OHCA-SPECIFIC POPULATION CHARACTERISTICS AND PREDICTORS OF MORTALITY

STEMI-induced CA is mostly related to ventricular fibrillation (VF). VF occurs at early stage of STEMI, and is most frequently out-of-hospital. This explains the importance of public access to defibrillation, which must be performed quickly in association with basic cardiac life support, followed by advanced cardiac life support on the basis of the European Resuscitation Council (ERC) guidelines for resuscitation.[13]

STEMI patients needing prehospital CPR are younger (64 years vs. 66 years) and more frequently have anterior STEMI or left bundle branch block (LBBB) compared with STEMI patients without prehospital CPR. Several factors have been identified as predictors of mortality: older age,[14] male gender,[14] asystole or pulseless electrical activity as initial heart rhythm,[10,15] unwitnessed events, need for epinephrine,[15] cardiac versus respiratory etiology of CA,[15] longer resuscitation time,[16] and longer time to return of spontaneous circulation (ROSC).[14] Predictors of mortality are important to optimize prehospital and hospital care, and to help determine the strategy of coronary reperfusion in both settings.

THROMBOLYSIS IN THE OHCA SETTING

The literature regarding thrombolysis for OHCA suffers from small-sample-size population, retrospective study designs, and lack of comparison of care and outcomes of STEMI patients with or without OHCA. On the basis of clinical reports, retrospective analysis, and some prospective studies, several studies demonstrated high survival rate and improved outcome when thrombolysis was given during CPR.[17,18] In contrast, in two large, randomized studies, no improvement of outcome was observed, although there was no increased incidence of bleeding.[7,9]

The use of fibrinolysis during CPR has to be considered in adult CA following initial CPR on a case-by-case basis when an acute thrombotic event is suspected. The patient with suspected pulmonary embolism is one example where thrombolysis can be considered. The ILCOR in 2005 recommended that "fibrinolysis should be considered in adult patients with CA with proven or suspected pulmonary embolism. There are insufficient data to support or refute the routine use of fibrinolysis in cardiac arrest from other causes."[12]

Safety Issues and Bleeding Risk

Several studies demonstrated the safety of thrombolytic therapy in patients with previous CPR.[7–9] When thrombolytic agents are used, CPR has to be continued for more than 60 to 90 minutes after administration. The European guidelines highlight that while a fibrinolytic agent is not contraindicated in successful CPR, it should be avoided in patients refractory to CPR. A meta-analysis pooling 8 studies assessing the fibrinolysis effect in CPR showed an increase rate of ROSC, 24-hour survival, discharge survival, and long-term neurologic function.[19] These results were not confirmed in the TROICA trial, which failed to demonstrate any beneficial effects of thrombolytic therapy.[20] In contrast, in the recent study by Koeth et al.,[21] the patients who received a thrombolytic agent as coronary reperfusion therapy demonstrated a significantly reduced in-hospital mortality (36.8% vs. 58.2% in the no-reperfusion group) in survivors of prehospital resuscitation with STEMI.

The risk of bleeding associated with thrombolytic therapy in the setting of OHCA has been a potential caution against the use of this therapy. Moreover, the routine use of fibrinolytics during CA has been demonstrated to increase the risk of intracranial bleeding.[20] In contrast, several studies with significant limitations demonstrated beneficial effects with improved outcome without any adverse events in terms of bleeding complications, especially no increased fibrinolysis-induced hemorrhagic complications, even when thrombolytic therapy was associated with heparin.[22] A lower rate of nonfatal stroke due to a preventive effect of brain microthrombi with fibrinolysis has been described.[23] Arntz et al.[4] recently demonstrated positive effects of targeted thrombolysis during CPR, confirming the results of previous studies on this beneficial effect of thrombolysis given to the right patient, at the right time, in the right condition.[4,17,18,19,22,24–28]

Although the data may be conflicting, the risks are still substantial enough that the indication for thrombolytic therapy during OHCA has to be considered on a case-by-case basis. The 2010 International Consensus on Cardiopulmonary Resuscitation and Emergency Cardiovascular Care Science with Treatment Recommendations reports that "routine administration of fibrinolytics for the treatment of in-hospital and out-of-hospital cardiac arrest is not recommended."[29]

ANGIOGRAPHY AND PPCI IN OHCA PATIENTS

Survivors of OHCA may benefit from mechanical coronary reperfusion as a result of PCI. Early cooling after CPR demonstrated beneficial effects with improved neurological outcomes in comatose patients who survived OHCA. Therapeutic hypothermia has to be instituted rapidly,[30,31] but the optimal delay between cooling and PPCI remains unclear. In all cases, angiography and/or PCI must not preclude or delay the strategy of therapeutic hypothermia.[32]

Some clinical events, such as presence of chest pain before CA, history of established coronary artery disease, and abnormal or doubtful ECG results that are signs of ongoing myocardial infarction, may be an indication for performing immediate angiography, as these events are related to potential coronary occlusions. Angiography may also have a role because of difficulties in interpretation of the ECG after CA. The ERC guidelines recommend performing a 12-lead ECG as soon as possible after ROSC. Different studies showed a high diagnostic reliability when ECGs are recorded during ongoing resuscitation (88% as reported by Arntz et al.[4]). Obtaining an ECG early on, even with unstable cardiocirculatory conditions, may still contribute to optimizing the therapy, particularly when a time-sensitive therapeutic option is considered.

The literature reports only a few studies on PPCI after OHCA. But it has been shown that coronary angiography and PCI were used as parts of a standardized, advanced post-CA protocol to reduce in-hospital mortality.[3,21,33] In a well-designed study, Lettieri et al.[16] reported that resuscitated OHCA patients who underwent emergency PCI for STEMI have a worse clinical presentation and a higher in-hospital mortality compared with patients without OHCA. However, subsequent cardiac events are similar, and neurologic recovery is more favorable than reported in most previous studies.[16] Coronary catheterization without PCI has been demonstrated to improve neurologic outcome.[34] One may keep in mind that a number of patients suffer from neurologic impairment before PCI. If this is the case, then the prognosis and beneficial effects from PCI in those patients remain unclear. Some small-sample-size studies suggested some beneficial effects.[3,5,35] Hosmane et al.[14] reported 92% full neurologic recovery in STEMI–OHCA survivors. In this nonrandomized study, predictors of survival were shorter ROSC, younger age, postresuscitation neurologic status alert or minimally responsive, and male sex.[14] Nevertheless, the outcome is better in short-duration, witnessed CA related to VF,[5,36] which underscores the beneficial effect of laypersons trained in CPR through the Public Access Defibrillation trial.[5,36] Better documentation of the predictors of neurologic recovery and overall survival may help guide future protocols and decisions regarding PCI after OHCA.

Is PCI Superior to Fibrinolysis?

Several studies[3,35,37] concluded that PCI seems to be more effective than thrombolysis in survivors of prehospital resuscitation with STEMI, if PCI can be performed as soon as possible. In some cases, PCI is lifesaving in OHCA patients who survived and presented with a STEMI diagnosis. So if PCI cannot be performed within 3 hours after CA onset, thrombolysis remains a good therapeutic strategy.

ADJUVANT THERAPIES FOR OHCA PATIENTS

The literature does not give any recommendations on the potential role of adjuvant antithrombotic and antiplatelet drugs, which remains to be explored in the case of OHCA–STEMI patients.[29]

CONCLUSION

A well-coordinated network between prehospital and hospital care must be established to offer STEMI–OHCA patients the best strategies within the best timeframe. Ongoing consultation between the emergency medical team and cardiologists, and the participation of the entire interprofessional cardiac acute care team will help to obtain the best outcome for these patients. As more data become available, specific protocols and educational programs for prehospital management of the OHCA–STEMI patient have to be developed.

REFERENCES

1. Holler NG, Mantoni T, Nielsen SL, Lippert F, Rasmussen LS. Long-term survival after out-of-hospital cardiac arrest. *Resuscitation.* 2007;75:23–28.
2. Zipes DP, Wellens HJ. Sudden cardiac death. *Circulation.* 1998;98:2334–2351.
3. Spaulding CM, Joly LM, Rosenberg A, et al. Immediate coronary angiography in survivors of out-of-hospital cardiac arrest. *N Engl J Med.* 1997;336:1629–1633.

4. Arntz HR, Wenzel V, Dissmann R, et al. Out-of-hospital thrombolysis during cardiopulmonary resuscitation in patients with high likelihood of ST-elevation myocardial infarction. *Resuscitation.* 2008;76:180–184.
5. Garot P, Lefevre T, Eltchaninoff H, et al. Six-month outcome of emergency percutaneous coronary intervention in resuscitated patients after cardiac arrest complicating ST-elevation myocardial infarction. *Circulation.* 2007;115:1354–1362.
6. Muller D, Schnitzer L, Brandt J, Arntz HR. The accuracy of an out-of-hospital 12-lead ECG for the detection of ST-elevation myocardial infarction immediately after resuscitation. *Ann Emerg Med.* 2008;52:658–664.
7. Van Campen LC, Van Leeuwen GR, Verheugt FW. Safety and efficacy of thrombolysis for acute myocardial infarction in patients with prolonged out-of-hospital cardiopulmonary resuscitation. *Am J Cardiol.* 1994;73:953–955.
8. Tenaglia AN, Califf RM, Candela RJ, et al. Thrombolysis therapy in patients requiring cardiopulmonary resuscitation. *Am J Cardiol.* 1991;68:1015–1019.
9. Scholtz KH, Tebbe U, Hermann C, et al. Frequency of complications of cardiopulmonary resuscitation after thrombolysis during acute myocardial infarction. *Am J Cardiol.* 1991;69:724–728.
10. Koeth O, Nibbe L, Arntz HR, et al. Fate of patients with prehospital resuscitation for ST-elevation myocardial infarction and a high rate of early reperfusion therapy (results from the PREMIR [Prehospital Myocardial Infarction Registry]). *Am J Cardiol.* 2012;109:1733–1737.
11. Engdahl J, Bang A, Karlson BW, et al. Long-term mortality among patients discharged alive after out-of-hospital cardiac arrest does not differ markedly compared with that of myocardial infarct patients without out-of-hospital cardiac arrest. *Eur J Emerg Med.* 2001;8:253–261.
12. International Liaison Committee on Resuscitation. 2005 International Consensus on Cardiopulmonary Resuscitation and Emergency Cardiovascular Care Science with Treatment Recommendations. Part 4. Advanced life support. *Resuscitation.* 2005;67:213–247.
13. ESC guidelines for the management of acute myocardial infarction in patients presenting with ST-segment elevation. *Eur Heart J.* 2012:33:2569–2619.
14. Hosmane VR, Mustafa NG, Reddy VK, et al. Survival and neurologic recovery in patients with ST-segment elevation myocardial infarction resuscitated from cardiac arrest. *J Am Coll Cardiol.* 2009;53:409–415.
15. Roberts D, Landolfo K, Light RB, Dobson K. Early predictors of mortality for hospitalized patients suffering cardiopulmonary arrest. *Chest.* 1990;97:413–415.

16. Lettieri C, Savonitto S, De Servi S, et al. Emergency percutaneous coronary intervention in patients with ST-elevation myocardial infarction complicated by out-of-hospital cardiac arrest: Early and medium-term outcome. *Am Heart J.* 2009;157:569–575.
17. Bottiger BW, Bode C, Kern S, et al. Efficacy and safety of thrombolytic therapy after initially unsuccessful cardiopulmonary resuscitation: A prospective clinical trial. *Lancet.* 2001;357:1583–1585.
18. Stadlbauer KH, Krismer AC, Arntz HR, et al. Effects of thrombolysis during out-of-hospital cardiopulmonary resuscitation. *Am J Cardiol.* 2006;97:305–308.
19. Li X, Fu QL, Jing XL, et al. A meta-analysis of cardiopulmonary resuscitation with and without the administration of thrombolytic agents. *Resuscitation.* 2006;70:31–36.
20. Bottiger BW, Arntz HR, Chamberlain DA. TROICA Trial Investigators: European Resuscitation Council Study Group. Thrombolysis during resuscitation for out-of-hospital cardiac arrest. *N Engl J Med.* 2008;359:2651–2662.
21. Koeth O, Zahn R, Bauer T, et al. Primary percutaneous coronary intervention and thrombolysis improve survival in patients with ST-elevation myocardial infarction and prehospital resuscitation. *Resuscitation.* 2010;81:1505–1508.
22. Riuz-Bailen M, Aguayo de Hoyos E, Serrano-Corcoles MC, et al. Efficacy of thrombolysis in patients with acute myocardial infarction requiring cardiopulmonary resuscitation. *Intensive Care Med.* 2001;27:1050–1057.
23. Fischer M, Bottiger BW, Popov-Cenic S, Hossmann KA. Thrombolysis using plasminogen-activator and heparin reduces cerebral no-reflow after resuscitation from cardiac arrest: An experimental study in the cat. *Intensive Care Med.* 1996;22:1214–1223.
24. Kurkciyan I, Meron G, Sterz F, et al. Major bleeding complications after cardiopulmonary resuscitation: impact of thrombolytic treatment. *J Intern Med.* 2003;253:128–135.
25. Lederer W, Lichtenberger C, Pechlaner C, Kroesen G, Baubin M. Recombinant tissue plasminogen activator during cardiopulmonary resuscitation in 108 patients with out-of-hospital cardiac arrest. *Resuscitation.* 2001;50:71–76.
26. Bozeman WP, Kleiner DM, Ferguson KL. Empiric tenecteplase is associated with increased return of spontaneous circulation and short term survival in cardiac arrest patients unresponsive to standard interventions. *Resuscitation.* 2006;69:399–406.
27. Fatovich DM, Dobb GJ, Clugston RA. A pilot randomized trial of thrombolysis in cardiac arrest (the TICA trial). *Resuscitation.* 2004;61:309–313.
28. Padosch SA, Motsch J, Bottiger BW. Thrombolysis during cardiopulmonary resuscitation. *Anaesthesist.* 2002;51:516–532.

29. Morrison LJ, Deakin CD, Morley PT, et al. 2010 International Consensus on Cardiopulmonary Resuscitation and Emergency Cardiovascular Care Science with Treatment Recommendations. Advanced Life Support; Part 8. *Circulation.* 2010;122(suppl 2):S345–S421.
30. Bernard SA, Gray TW, Buist MD, et al. Treatment of comatose survivors of out-of-hospital cardiac arrest with induced hypothermia. *N Engl J Med.* 2002;346:549–556.
31. Belliard G, Catez E, Charron C, et al. Efficacy of therapeutic hypothermia after 2out-of-hospital cardiac arrest due to ventricular fibrillation. *Resuscitation.* 2007;75:252–259.
32. O'Connor R, Brady W, Brooks SC, et al. Acute coronary syndromes: 2010 American Heart Association guidelines for cardiopulmonary resuscitation and emergency cardiovascular care. Part 10. *Circulation.* 2010;122:S787–S817.
33. Sunde K, Pytte M, Jacobsen D, et al. Implementation of a standardised treatment protocol for post resuscitation care after out-of-hospital cardiac arrest. *Resuscitation.* 2007;73:29–39.
34. Reynolds JC, Callaway CW, El Khoudary, et al. Coronary angiography predicts improved outcome following cardiac arrest: propensity-adjusted analysis. *J Intensive Care Med.* 2009;24:179–186.
35. McCullogh PA, Prakash R, Tobin KJ, O'Neill WW, Thompson RJ. Application of a cardiac arrest score in patients with sudden death and ST segment elevation for triage to angiography and intervention. *J Interv Cardiol.* 2002;15:257–261.
36. Gorjup V, Radsel P, Kocjancic ST, Erzen D, Noc M. Acute ST-elevation myocardial infarction after successful cardiopulmonary resuscitation. *Resuscitation.* 2007;72:379–385.
37. Keelan PC, Bunch TJ, White RD, Packer DL, Holmes DR. Early direct coronary angioplasty in survivors of out-of-hospital cardiac arrest. *Am J Cardiol.* 2003;1461–1463.

CHAPTER 7

Role of Nurses and Paramedics in the Prehospital Care of Acute Myocardial Infarction

Denise Greci Robinson, RN, MS, CNS

INTRODUCTION

A well-trained and organized emergency medical services (EMS) system is critical to the recognition, triage, and treatment of acute ST-elevation myocardial infarction (STEMI) and non-ST elevation myocardial infarction (NSTEMI). Time to reperfusion can be divided into four phases: (1) the onset of patient's symptoms; (2) the patient actively seeks treatment by activating EMS or traveling to a medical facility by private vehicle; (3) initiation of reperfusion therapies which may be administered in the prehospital phase; and (4) emergent revascularization hospital care with percutaneous coronary intervention (PCI). In each phase, nurses and paramedics (emergency medical personnel with advanced training and certifications) provide specialized knowledge and skillful practice to initiate treatment and reduce delays to reperfusion that are integral to achieving better outcomes for patients. Therefore, the purpose of this chapter is to review barriers

Prehospital Management of Acute STEMI: Practical Approaches and International Strategies for Early Intervention © 2015 Joseph S. Alpert, Lynne T. Braun, Barbara J. Fletcher, Gerald Fletcher, Editors-in-Chief, Cardiotext Publishing, ISBN: 978-1-935395-66-9

to early recognition of acute coronary syndrome (ACS), the role of paramedics and nurses in optimizing interventions and system processes, and outcome measurement to improve systematic care.

GUIDELINES FOR ACHIEVING OPTIMAL OUTCOMES

The 2013 American College of Cardiology Foundation/American Heart Association (ACCF/AHA) STEMI guidelines recommend that systems of care are developed to increase the number of patients with timely access to primary percutaneous coronary intervention (PPCI).[1] These guidelines recommend that the first medical contact-to-balloon time be within 90 minutes or less for patients presenting to a PCI capable hospital. For those patients who initially present to a non-PCI-capable hospital, the guideline is to transfer the patient to a PCI-capable hospital and achieve balloon inflation within 120 minutes or less from the first medical contact. Research has shown that door-to-balloon times are achieved more often when patients are identified in the field and transported directly to a designated center for PCI than when patients are evaluated by physicians in emergency departments (EDs) of non-PCI-capable hospitals.[2,3] Patients who present to a non-PCI-capable hospital and are transferred for PCI have a statistically significant higher mortality rate than those who present directly from the field to a PCI center.[4] Nurses and paramedics are in a position to optimize interventions and system processes during this time frame from first medical contact to guideline-based therapy.

BARRIERS TO TREATMENT

There can be no treatment without recognition. Chest pain is one of the most common and complex symptoms for which patients seek emergency medical care; however, there are barriers that delay a person's time to seek treatment. A patient's presenting symptoms may differ from the historical bias that a heart attack should present dramatically with classic crushing chest pain; this often leads to a delay in seeking treatment. Delay from time of symptom onset to actively seeking treatment can be related to a lack of knowledge of heart attack symptoms, maladaptive coping strategies, or misattribution of symptoms to a potentially less serious cause.[5-11] Prehospital delay has been shown to be longer among several populations: women longer than men, non-Hispanic blacks longer than non-Hispanic whites, longer at older ages, and longer among Medicaid-only recipients.[8]

ROLE OF THE PARAMEDIC IN REDUCING THE PREHOSPITAL DELAY TO TREATMENT OF ACS

Prehospital delay has been shown to be shorter in patients who used an ambulance for transportation. Unfortunately, patients with STEMI often do not utilize emergency services for transport to the hospital. In a 2011 observational study using US data, from the ACTION Registry Get With the Guidelines, only 60% of 37,643 patients presenting with STEMI used the EMS transport.[9] This disparity needs to be addressed by public health and educational initiatives centered on identifying one's risk factors for ACS and recognition of typical and atypical symptoms. Paramedics and nurses are ideally suited to provide public outreach and education on this as well as emphasize the importance of activating EMS.

For patients who activate EMS, the paramedic provider is in a position of rapidly eliciting a history, completing a physical assessment, performing diagnostic testing, and initiating lifesaving interventions. These activities can improve outcomes by identifying ACS early and facilitating triage and transport to a facility capable of intervention. Thus, the paramedic provider needs to have knowledge of the typical and atypical presentations of ACS and quickly run through the differential diagnosis related to chest pain. The prehospital provider should solicit and record a history that includes the character of pain by considering specific aspects of the history such as onset, severity, quality, location, radiation, frequency, duration, precipitating or mitigating factors, relationship to exertion, and response to therapy. The paramedic should then assess for any associated symptoms such as shortness of breath, dyspnea on exertion, paroxysmal nocturnal dyspnea, nausea, vomiting, diaphoresis, cough, sputum production, hemoptysis, fever, chills, fatigue, dizziness, syncope, and palpitations. The provider should also solicit information from the patient's past medical history that implies risk factors for coronary artery disease (CAD) as well as possible recent illness, medications, recent surgery or procedures, recent diagnostic testing, and substance abuse. The physical examination should consist of vital signs including pulse oximetry, assessment of respiratory rate and effort, auscultation of lungs, palpation of pulse for quality and regularity, and assessment of skin signs, noting any pallor, diaphoresis, or edema.

On the basis of the history and the physical assessment thus far, the paramedic can direct interventions accordingly. During transport, several interventions provided by paramedic personnel can be lifesaving and will save time once the patient arrives at the receiving facility. Chapter 2 provides a detailed discussion of adjunctive prehospital pharmacotherapy for this purpose. For the patient with chest pain suggestive of cardiac origin, the paramedic should perform a 12-lead ECG. It is at this critical point that EMS agencies can differ significantly in their capabilities and protocols.

ROLE OF PREHOSPITAL ECG PERFORMED BY PARAMEDICS

Some EMS agencies have paramedics perform prehospital ECGs. Research has demonstrated that this intervention reduces the time delay from the decision to seek treatment to diagnosis.[12-14] For an EMS early STEMI recognition system to be successful, the first-responding clinicians need to have the training and equipment necessary to independently make the triage decision. The difficulty in standardizing this training across regions with a range of resources has been discussed in detail in previous chapters.

For some patients, the ECG may not be diagnostic, and therefore the paramedic will need to rely on the presentation of the patient and the history and physical assessment. Research investigating prehospital point-of-care (POC) testing for cardiac biomarkers of myocardial necrosis has also been conducted. One study looked at the reliability of POC for cardiac troponin I (cTnI) on the ambulance during transport and found that the results on the ambulance highly correlated to the results obtained when the POC testing devices were used in ED.[15] While more research is needed to validate these findings as well as to look at the feasibility, practicality, and clinical utility of prehospital use of POC testing devices, this type of intervention could reduce the time delay to diagnosis and reperfusion by utilizing the transport time to perform testing.

PREHOSPITAL THROMBOLYTIC THERAPY

Although reperfusion through PPCI is the preferred mode of reperfusion therapy, in many areas of the United States there is a limited access to PCI-capable centers. Interfacility or prehospital transport to medical facilities capable of performing PCI or administering fibrinolytics can cause delays in reperfusion. Prehospital fibrinolysis, which helps reduce the total ischemic time, is an important treatment consideration.[16-18] Most EMS systems in the United States do not have teams trained in the administration of prehospital fibrinolysis. However, in some areas after paramedics identify STEMI patients and provide initial interventions, protocols are initiated to assess a patient's eligibility for thrombolytic therapy and provide that treatment. Chapter 2 offers a more complete discussion of this topic.

ROLE OF NURSES IN PREHOSPITAL MANAGEMENT OF ACS

The role of the nurse in the management of the acute infarct patient is multifaceted, ranging from direct patient care in the ED setting and during interfacility transport, to program development, performance improvement, research, and policy making. All nurses are trained in the nursing process, a modified scientific method composed of the elements of assessment, diagnosis, outcomes/planning, implementation, and evaluation. Through education and training as well as practical experience, this process of critical thinking becomes the foundation for nursing assessments and interventions. Thus, nursing process is highly relevant for designing and evaluating systems of prehospital STEMI care.

Direct Patient Care

Nurses are involved in assessment and triage of patients that present to ED, whether by private vehicle or by EMS transport. The nurse is often the first point of medical contact at the hospital and as such must possess the skills to perform an initial assessment and identify the need for further and timely diagnostic testing. Much the same as paramedics, emergency nurses must be able to take a pertinent history and physical assessment to gather the information necessary to work through the differential diagnosis for chest pain. Depending on the facility, nurses may initiate protocols to begin treatment of patients prior to a physician seeing the patient. These protocols include interventions such as obtaining a 12-lead ECG, gaining IV access, drawing and ordering laboratory tests, ordering a chest x-ray, initiating sublingual nitroglycerine and aspirin administration. In most centers with STEMI protocols, the timeframe goal for door-of-ED to ECG is 10 minutes. The ED nurse is paramount to meeting this goal.

The role of the critical care transport nurse (CCT RN) is to transport critically ill patients from one medical facility to another for a higher level of care. In many areas, the CCT RN is trained in central and arterial line insertion and monitoring, advanced airway management, management of intraaortic balloon pumps, and other critical care procedures. These nurses are highly trained and have advanced certifications to perform this role. These nurses utilize a higher fund of knowledge to assess and diagnose critically ill patients than that of the paramedic provider. Their knowledge and skill set paired with paramedic and or EMS providers affords the level of care necessary for interfacility transport of the critically ill STEMI patient.

Program Development

Nurses can assess the needs of the community and the particular patient population that they serve by evaluating the current state of STEMI care at their hospital, county, and state. The nurse can help to identify and resolve barriers to improving outcomes both at the hospital level as well as the county or EMS system level. The nurse can take into account the current resources, stakeholders, and financial considerations. Utilizing their specialized research education and training as well as clinical knowledge base, nurses can then develop solutions to address the barriers to meeting predetermined goals and achieving the best possible outcomes for patients. Nurses do this on large and small levels. For example, the emergency nurse notices that her department is not meeting door-to-ECG goals and identifies the need for more ECG machines and/or delays in the triage process, lack of organization in the pre-treatment area, need for ancillary staff, and so forth. The nurse then utilizes evidence-based practice and research to develop solutions and programs to address the issues.

Advanced practice nurses such as clinical nurse specialists (CNS) and nurse practitioners (NP) often have important positions within the interprofessional team for STEMI care. At the same time, they are specially trained in research utilization and program development, making them the ideal practitioners to collaborate with physician and EMS colleagues to develop STEMI programs at the hospital and community level. This requires collaboration between local EMS, nurses in the catheterization laboratory (CL), cardiologists, ED physicians and nurses, as well as hospital administration. A successful program first requires research into current guidelines and best practice. Implementation requires a tremendous amount of education of stakeholders and staff as well as coordination among all services involved. Nurse managers are in a position to implement and facilitate the recommendations from the STEMI program by providing their bedside nurses with the resources required to meet the needs of the program and make the necessary changes. This may include assessing and adjusting staffing, seeking out and providing the needed equipment, and providing for and supporting additional education for the program components.

Evaluation and Outcome Measurement

Any successful performance improvement project must have a framework to organize the steps of the project, keeping in mind that performance improvement is cyclical. The PDCA cycle is a methodology often used, and the acronym stands for Plan-Do-Check-Act or Plan-Do-Check-Adjust. In the planning phase of the project, the objectives are established including the expected outcomes. For example, the objective of reducing door-to-balloon time for STEMI patients arriving by ambulance to a particular hospital by at least 10 minutes from a previous 90-minute timeframe would be established in the "Plan" stage. Then, the necessary processes or steps to create the change would need to be identified. The next stage is "Do," where the plan is implemented. In this example, the plan may include implementing automatic transmission of a prehospital ECG and initiating code STEMI activation from the field ECG for a positive transmission. The next stage is "Check," where measured and collected data is analyzed and compared with expected results or targets from the "Plan." Keeping with the current example, pertinent data would include false-positive and false-negative CL activations, technical difficulties encountered, time of ED arrival to departure for CL, door-to-balloon times, and EMS encounter-to-balloon times. Once information is analyzed, and strengths and weaknesses are identified, then it is time to "Adjust or Act" on the significant differences between the actual and planned results. Efforts at this point can be targeted to specific areas of the plan that are ineffective or identified as problem areas. From this point, one would return to the planning stage with more specific, targeted goals and identify process steps necessary to meet those goals. Nurses and paramedic providers can utilize this framework in their respective roles as they care for the acute infarct patient. Whether they are involved in program development on a larger systems scale or in direct patient care, once goals are identified, this framework can be utilized to work toward achieving the best possible outcome for patients. Nurses and paramedics teach basic life support (BLS) and advanced cardiac life support (ACLS), and hold leadership roles in the American Heart Association's Mission: Lifeline program. They are also active on state advocacy committees, where they lobby for coordinated and effective STEMI systems of care.

CONCLUSION

Paramedic providers and nurses work within their respective scope of practice to improve the care of the acute infarct patient. They are specially trained to provide direct care ensuring that patients are properly assessed, treated, triaged, and transported to receive the most effective reperfusion therapy. Both paramedics and nurses hold positions in the community that allow for direct access to populations that would benefit from outreach and education related to the signs and symptoms of myocardial infarction (MI) as well as the importance of activating EMS for help and transportation. On a systems level, advanced practice nurses are especially suited to integrate their knowledge of research utilization and evidence-based practice to work with their hospital and EMS colleagues to develop successful STEMI programs in both a hospital and regional setting. Any successful program will have a framework of continuous performance improvement and outcome evaluation.

REFERENCES

1. O'Gara PT, Kuschner FG, Ascheim DD, et al. 2013 ACCF/AHA guideline for the management of ST-elevation myocardial infarction: executive summary: a report on the American College of Cardiology Foundation/American Heart Association task force on practice guidelines. *Circulation*. 2013;127(4):529–555.
2. Bradley EH, Herrin J, Wang Y, et al. Strategies for reducing the door-to-balloon time in acute myocardial infarction. *N Engl J Med*. 2006;355:2308–2320.
3. Le May MR, So DY, Dionne R, et al. A citywide protocol for primary PCI in ST-segment elevation myocardial infarction. *N Engl J Med*. 2008;358:231–240.
4. Le May MR, Wells GA, So DY, et al. Reduction in mortality as a result of direct transport from the field to a receiving center for primary percutaneous coronary intervention. *J Am Coll Cardiol*. 2012;60(14):1223–1230.
5. Goff DC, Feldman HA, McGovern PG, et al. Prehospital delay in patients hospitalized with heart attack symptoms in the United States: The REACT trial. *Am Heart J*. 1999;138(6):1046–1057.

6. Mathews R, Peterson ED, Li S, et al. Use of emergency medical service transport among patients with ST-segment–elevation myocardial infarction findings from the national cardiovascular data registry acute coronary treatment intervention outcomes network registry–get with the guidelines. *Circulation.* 2011;124:154–163.
7. Brieger D, Eagle KA, Goodman SG, et al. Acute coronary syndromes without chest pain, an underdiagnosed and undertreated high-risk group: insights from the Global Registry of Acute Coronary Events. *Chest.* 2004;126:461–469.
8. Bleeker JK, Lamers LM, Leenders IM, et al. Psychological and knowledge factors related to delay of help-seeking by patients with acute myocardial infarction. *Psychother Psychosom.* 1995;63:151–158.
9. Meischke H, Eisenberg MS, Schaeffer SM, et al. Utilization of emergency medical services for symptoms of acute myocardial infarction. *Heart Lung.* 1995;24:11–18.
10. Meischke H, Ho MT, Eisenberg MS, et al. Reasons patients with chest pain delay or do not call 911. *Ann Emerg Med.* 1995;25:193–197.
11. Johnson JA, King KB. Influence of expectations about symptoms on delay in seeking treatment during a myocardial infarction. *Am J Crit Care.* 1995;4:29–35.
12. Ting HH, Krumholz HM, Bradley EH, et al. Implementation and integration of prehospital ECGs into systems of care for acute coronary syndrome. A scientific statement from the American Heart Association Interdisciplinary Council on Quality of Care and Outcomes Research, Emergency Cardiovascular Care Committee, Council on Cardiovascular Nursing, and Council on Clinical Cardiology. *Cardiology.* 2008;118:1066–1079.
13. Le May MR, So DY, Dionne R, et al. A citywide protocol for primary PCI in ST-segment elevation myocardial infarction. *N Engl J Med.* 2008;358:231–240.
14. Jollis JG, Roettig ML, Aluko AO, et al. Implementation of a statewide system for coronary reperfusion for ST-segment elevation myocardial infarction. *JAMA.* 2007;298:2371–2380.
15. Venturini JM, Stake CE, Cichon ME. Prehospital point-of-care testing for troponin: are the results reliable? *Prehosp Emerg Care.* 2013;17(1)88–91.
16. Antman EM. Time is muscle. *J Am Coll Cardiol.* 2008;52(15)1216–1221.
17. Bonnefoy E, Lapostolle F, Leizorovicz A, et al. Primary angioplasty versus prehospital fibrinolysis in acute myocardial infarction: a randomized study. *Lancet.* 2002;360:825–829.
18. Steg PG, Bonnefoy E, Chabaud S, et al. Impact of time to treatment on mortality after prehospital fibrinolysis or primary angioplasty: Data from the CAPTIM randomized clinical trial. *Circulation.* 2003;108:2851–2856.

Part 2

Systems of Prehospital STEMI Care from Around the World

CHAPTER 8

Canada: Integrated Systems of Prehospital STEMI Care

Darren Knapp, EMT-P, and Robert C. Welsh, MD

EPIDEMIOLOGY AND GEOGRAPHIC REALITIES IN CANADA

Occupying the upper half of the continent of North America, Canada, known for the diversity of its people and their cultures, is an expansive land mass and the second largest country in the world (over 9,984,000 km^2 or 3,854,000 square miles). However, with a population of approximately 35 million in 2012, Canada has a relatively low population density of approximately 3.4 inhabitants/km^2; although roughly 80% of the population occupy large urban cities, typically within 150 km of the largest international land border between Canada and the United States (8900 km or 5525 miles). Canada's wide-stretching, sparsely populated rural areas present a unique challenge to deliver effective and timely acute myocardial infarction (AMI) care to all citizens, especially from an Emergency Medical Services (EMS) standpoint.

In Canada, death from heart disease is the second leading cause of death in both males and females, with over 16,000 Canadians dying each year as the result of a heart attack. There are an estimated 70,000 heart attacks each year in Canada, with one heart attack occurring every 7 minutes. Most of these deaths occur prior to the patient's arrival to a hospital.

Prehospital Management of Acute STEMI: Practical Approaches and International Strategies for Early Intervention © 2015 Joseph S. Alpert, Lynne T. Braun, Barbara J. Fletcher, Gerald Fletcher, Editors-in-Chief, Cardiotext Publishing, ISBN: 978-1-935395-66-9

The economic burden of heart disease is substantial, with the number of heart attack-related hospitalizations increasing steadily over the past decade (1994–95 to 2003–04).[1]

TERTIARY HEALTHCARE ACCESS IN CANADA

The federal government provides national healthcare policies and with few exceptions, it is a publicly funded healthcare system. The country is divided into 10 provinces and 3 territories, and the legislation and administration of health care rests at the provincial level. This funding model provides the backbone budgeting necessary to implement systems of care, including prehospital EMS, primary care, care in community, and tertiary hospitals that must collaborate to optimize patient management. In contrast to comparable nations, Canada has relatively few tertiary care centers with capacity to deliver invasive cardiac catheterization and percutaneous coronary intervention (PCI), and these tertiary care centers are only present in the country's major urban centers. Across the country, there are approximately 45 tertiary care centers with the capacity to conduct cardiac catheterization and 24/7 primary percutaneous coronary intervention (PPCI). The three northern territories and one province (Prince Edward Island) have no cardiac catheterization facilities. It has been previously established that approximately 65% of Canadians aged 40 years and older had access to a PCI facility within 60 minutes.[2]

PREHOSPITAL STEMI MANAGEMENT SYSTEMS IN CANADA

Within the public model of health care, the Emergency Medical Systems (EMS) in Canada are as diverse as the geography and culture. Primarily there are 2 dominant models of operational and administrative systems for EMS: either a publicly administered system or a privately owned and operated ambulance service. Public sector services are government-funded EMS that are administered and operated directly by government-based healthcare systems at the municipal, regional, or provincial level. Privately owned and operated EMS often enter into contracts with the provincial or territorial government to provide EMS coverage on behalf of the provincial healthcare system. While private services are enterprising capital ventures, often they are legislated and contractually bound to provide care according to the medical direction and guideline policies outlined by the provincial healthcare body. This hybrid of direct public and privately contracted services is featured in provinces such as Alberta under the provincial healthcare system, Alberta Health Services (AHS).

Across the country, a public 911 phone system directs calls to a Public Safety Access Point where the need is determined for police services, fire services, and/or EMS. Patient care that is delivered by EMS in the community is guided using a physician-driven medical direction model, which is a hybrid of what is known as "online and offline" medical direction. Offline medical direction provides EMS with a standing-order set of protocols or guidelines to follow, and these outline the standard of care to be delivered by the EMS practitioners in most emergent situations. An "online" component is added to support the offline model, where EMS can or must call in and speak to an on-call medical director or predefined physician for further advice on specific advanced therapies.

LEVELS OF PREHOSPITAL EMS CARE-PROVIDERS

There are 2 major categorical levels of prehospital care delivery across most of Canada: basic life support (BLS) and advanced life support (ALS). These levels are divided into professional designations that include the emergency medical responder (EMR) and primary care paramedic (PCP) under a BLS system, and the advanced care paramedic (ACP), and critical care paramedic (CCP) for the ALS system. These practitioner levels of competency are defined by a scope of practice, and describe the care that can be delivered and the skills that each level can bring to emergencies such as cardiac arrest. Several provinces have a professional college for EMS practitioners where they must be registered to provide EMS care, and do so under a combination of online and offline medical oversights. These professional colleges oversee the registration, scope of practice, discipline, and licensure of practitioners separate from their employers, be it public or private services. Exclusive to the province of Quebec, which has a BLS-based prehospital system, there are a limited number of prehospital ambulance units that have a physician in the prehospital environment.

STRATEGIES FOR PREHOSPITAL STEMI CARE: A GRADUATED APPROACH

In Canada, there are nearly an equal percentage of STEMI patients that present via EMS and that "walk-in" direct to an emergency department (ED), with higher usage of EMS in urban environments and lower usage in the rural setting. Not all EMS systems are alike in their approach to prehospital STEMI, as medical directors in concert with local cardiology-based systems of care often dictate how in-depth a reperfusion strategy can be. When EMS practitioners are the point of first medical contact with a patient, decisions regarding treatment of STEMI are first dictated by offline protocol, followed by any specialized regional approaches to AMI care in that area. We outline the framework for the 5 steps in prehospital care that represent a graduated approach to achieving timely reperfusion therapy within the Canadian healthcare system. As might be expected, the latter steps require more access to trained personnel and tertiary care centers and are not as widely available as the earlier steps.

Patient Screening

STEMI care from a BLS standpoint often involves a general patient assessment, history taking, and the acquisition of basic vital signs. Education for prehospital providers focuses on typical symptom recognition (chest, jaw, or shoulder pain or discomfort), key history interview questions related to the qualities of the pain or discomfort that the patient is experiencing, and practitioners are warned to be highly suspicious of anginal equivalents (weakness, dizziness, shortness of breath, etc.). In addition to these techniques and findings, EMS crews are also asked to consider other risk factors or links that point to cardiac disease, such as family history and lifestyle risk factors, to complete the clinical picture.

Acquiring a 12-lead ECG

The capacity to acquire a prehospital 12-lead ECG is variable across Canada, available in the majority of urban centers (estimated 70% of the urban population) but far less predictable in the rural communities (estimated 30% of the rural population). There is significant intraprovincial variation ranging from 40% in Quebec to 100% in Alberta and Nova Scotia.[3] For certain levels of practitioners, their scope of practice will include the ability to acquire a 12-lead ECG (PCPs), although advanced ECG interpretation for differentiating STEMI is not undertaken at this level. Higher-trained ALS practitioners (ACPs, CCP, or emergency medical technologist-paramedic) are capable of acquiring an ECG and conducting preliminary or advanced interpretation. As most ALS systems rely on combination of one BLS and one ALS level practitioner working together as a team, the BLS providers provide the key clinical support to what becomes a very busy patient case to manage. The prehospital care environment is a compelling example of collaborative efficiency in optimal situations with BLS providers establishing intravenous access, giving oral doses of aspirin (ASA), and potentially nitroglycerin.

In rural Canada where strictly BLS EMS systems are in the majority, transfer to the nearest hospital remains the standard of care. This presents an obvious challenge in delivering time-dependent critical reperfusion therapies for STEMI to rural Canadians. Not only does this increase the time of infarct according to the distance needed to travel to seek ALS support, but the BLS practitioners' scope of practice does not allow them to provide fibrinolysis or even early antithrombotic and antiplatelet therapies outside of ASA. Once an ALS level practitioner is available to assist, the 12-lead ECG is reviewed for suspicious ST-segment deviation and further care steps can be taken. Typically, a second ambulance unit from a larger community with ALS care support arrives as back up, or alternatively definitive diagnosis awaits arrival at the nearest hospital ED.

Prehospital Checklists and Offline Treatment Algorithms for BLS and ALS Paramedics

The development of prehospital STEMI checklists is of paramount importance to the standardized approach to the diagnosis, risk stratification, and treatment of this disease. They allow for the rapid identification of key steps in care, and serve as prompts to ensure that critical history and clinical issues are adequately addressed in determining reperfusion strategies. Checklists typically include baseline clinical vital signs, hemodynamic status, critical review of ECG criteria, timelines related to the onset of symptoms, and clinical care benchmarks with review for eligibility to receive fibrinolysis by using key indications and contraindications.

Offline protocols can include directions on antiplatelet therapy, management of hypotension, arrhythmia management, and resuscitation guidelines for associated cardiac arrest. The EMS crew often works in concert with each other and with concurrent protocols to cover all aspects of care prior to seeking a reperfusion decision. ALS practitioners (ACP, PCP) have an expanded skill set, which builds on the BLS platform and allows for advanced arrhythmia detection and management, enhanced medication profiles, and 12-lead and 15-lead ECG interpretation essential to STEMI recognition and AMI care.

Additionally, in some areas, offline protocols may include criteria for triage of potential STEMI patients to tertiary care PCI centers with bypass of community hospitals when operating within a defined STEMI system of care. These EMS systems in Canada will direct suspected ACS/STEMI patients to ED of a tertiary care center following preliminary ECG interpretation. Conversely, several systems in major centers will actually bypass the ED and transport directly to the cardiac catheterization laboratory where a STEMI diagnosis can be made, and urgent or emergent PCI can be performed.

Within Canada this process of using offline protocols to triage prehospital STEMI patients has been shown to effectively reduce treatment delays and improve time to PPCI and has become the standard approach in the majority of urban centers. In metropolitan Ottawa, Ontario, paramedic-based prehospital offline STEMI diagnosis and triage direct to the PPCI center was associated with a 91-minute time from ECG to first balloon inflation (91 median, interquartile range [IQR]: 66–113 minutes), which was 17 minutes faster than in patients undergoing interhospital transfer (108 median, IQR: 91–129 minutes).[4] Similarly in metropolitan Calgary, Alberta, this approach achieved a median time from EMS arrival on scene to coronary reperfusion of 97 minutes (median, IQR: 76–124 minutes).[5]

Online Support for Early EMS Diversion to Tertiary Care PCI Centers or Fibrinolysis in the ED

Physician directed online support for paramedic triage decisions requires the crucial step of 12-lead ECG acquisition and transmission to confirm the diagnosis of STEMI. ECG transmission systems often involve third-party vendors with software and infrastructure developed to facilitate secure, cellular, or internet-based transmission of the ECG data.

In communities that offer ALS-based models, STEMI recognition is undertaken by the attending EMS paramedic crew with ECG transmission to a local ED, direct to an ECG work station in the cardiac catheterization center or to a mobile device for physician review. This modality of detection and consultation facilitates triage and timeliness of in-hospital reperfusion therapy. This is especially true when PPCI is sought or preferred over a fibrinolytic approach. In major urban centers, this is often the case, and this same system of care can often be extended to include suburban and even rural EMS services within a reasonable transportation radius. In this type of system, fibrinolysis may be preferred in appropriately selected patients, but this scenario requires the rural EMS crew to transport to the nearest ED, ideally with prehospital activation to deliver pharmacological reperfusion immediately upon hospital arrival. Unfortunately, further physician review, repeat ECGs, and consultation may delay initiation of reperfusion therapy. Following fibrinolysis, various protocols have been developed to transfer the patient, be it by ground or by air, to the nearest site capable of performing rescue PCI in the event of a failure of the fibrinolysis.

The addition of prehospital 12-lead ECG transmission has been shown to further decrease treatment delays. In metropolitan Winnipeg, Manitoba, this approach achieved a time from first medical contact to PPCI of 76 minutes (median76, IQR: 64–93 minutes), which represents 20 to 30 minutes of additional reduction in treatment delay.[6,7]

Fully Integrated Systems for ED Bypass to PCI and/or Prehospital Fibrinolysis—Dual-Reperfusion Therapy Systems in Canada

Previous investigations have demonstrated that paramedics-based prehospital fibrinolysis is feasible and applicable operating within such a fully integrated STEMI system.[8] Additionally, there was no treatment delay or increased patient risk demonstrated of paramedic compared with physician-based prehospital fibrinolysis.[9]

The recently published Strategic Reperfusion Early After Myocardial Infarction (STREAM) study, previously discussed in Chapter 2, supports the benefit of a dedicated dual-reperfusion strategy.[9] In this study, which randomized patients presenting within 3 hours of symptom onset to prehospital fibrinolysis or expedited PPCI within established STEMI systems of care, fibrinolysis with tenecteplase was associated with a 30-day composite event rate (death, repeat myocardial infarction [MI], heart failure, and shock) of 12.4% in the fibrinolysis group, which compared favorably with expedited PPCI of 14.3% (relative risk reduction, 0.86; 95% confidence interval, 0.68–1.09; $P = 0.21$).

In a limited number of ALS services in Canada, fully integrated dual-reperfusion therapy is already available within a comprehensive system of STEMI care (Figure 8.1) that uses both the offline and online approaches. In a typical scenario, EMS ALS ambulances will conduct patient assessments, 12-lead ECG preliminary interpretation and use offline protocols to achieve a preliminary diagnosis and assess reperfusion criteria. Then, other components of the fully integrated system are implemented in an interprofessional team approach that combines all of the aforementioned elements incorporating

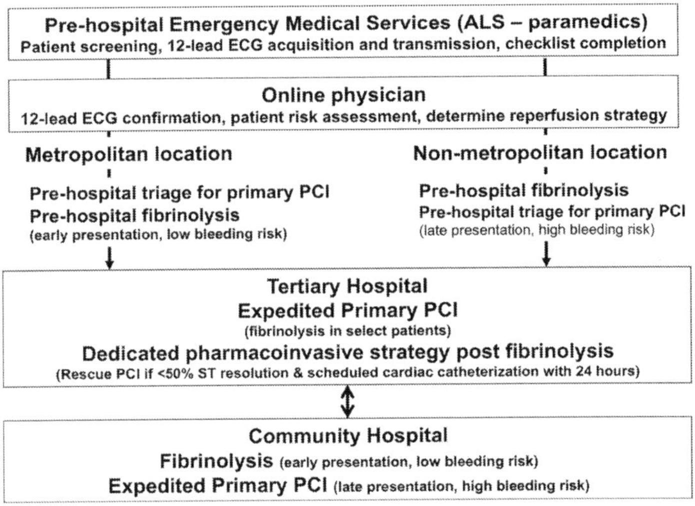

Figure 8.1

Contemporary management of STEMI according to dual reperfusion. An optimal STEMI reperfusion program integrates the tertiary PPCI hospital with prehospital EMS, interhospital transfer, and community hospitals without the capacity for PPCI. Individual patients are assessed at the point of presentation including dedicated prehospital diagnosis and triage. That patient reperfusion decision is based upon time from symptoms onset, baseline clinical characteristics, estimated bleeding risks and informed predicted time to reperfusion therapy. The expected use of pharmacological or mechanical reperfusion is presented in sequence in the figure, which acknowledges where the patient presented: ambulance or hospital, community or tertiary hospital, and metropolitan or nonmetropolitan region.

ALS prehospital teams, an ECG transmission system, offline and online medical control, and the ability to advance the reperfusion decision upstream into the EMS environment. One such example of a fully integrated system is the Vital Heart Response protocol in Central and Northern Alberta. In this system, in consultation with a dedicated physician team, each case and key data, including the ECG and presenting clinical characteristics, is reviewed and reperfusion decisions are weighed accordingly. Full medical therapy with evidence-based prehospital antithrombin and antiplatelet therapies and direct transport to the cardiac catheterization laboratory for PPCI, bypassing community hospitals and the tertiary care ED, is used in approximately 70% of urban and suburban STEMI patients.[10] Additionally, if the optimal reperfusion strategy is deemed to be fibrinolytics, which occurs in approximately 30% of urban patients, reperfusion therapy is administered in the ambulance with evidence-based adjunctive antithrombotic and antiplatelet therapy and subsequently transported to facilitate assessment of reperfusion success and rescue PCI or routine cardiac catheterization within a dedicated pharmacoinvasive approach. In the rural environment, fibrinolysis is used in the majority (approximately 60%) of patients with PPCI only used in late-presenting patients or those with perceived excessive bleeding risk. In situations where prolonged transportation is required following fibrinolytic therapy, EMS ALS crews routinely repeat the 12-lead ECG in transit and can active the cardiac catheterization laboratory directly from the ambulance for rescue PCI in the setting of reperfusion failure.

This fully integrated system of care with dual-reperfusion strategies is associated with only a 16% rate of failure to receive reperfusion therapy and has shown improved outcomes for STEMI patients with significantly lower risk-adjusted rates for 30-day mortality compared with other regions within Canada.[1] In addition, the dual-reperfusion strategy bridges the gap between nonmetropolitan and metropolitan STEMI patients. Specifically, within a comprehensive dual-reperfusion STEMI system, a dedicated pharmacoinvasive approach is associated with similar outcomes for nonmetropolitan patients compared with metropolitan patient who receive PPCI the majority of the time (death, reinfarction, heart failure, cardiogenic shock: nonmetropolitan 15.1% compared with metropolitan 16.8%, $P = 0.161$).[10,11] This is especially relevant in nations such as Canada that have substantial geographic challenges and large rural areas.

CONCLUSION

Globally, the burden of cardiovascular disease is extensive. Implementing interprofessional teams of prehospital management of AMI represents a key priority and opportunity to improve patient outcomes. Nationally and regionally there are unique cultural, financial, and geographical challenges that must be incorporated into development of STEMI systems of care. Acknowledging these variations, the successful impact of dedicated STEMI reperfusion systems provides compelling evidence that mandates investment into program development and refinement. The challenge that Canada faces is providing equal access to all patients under a publicly funded health system while providing top-line therapies to all, given the large geographic area that it encompasses.

Therefore, it is crucial to integrate a multidisciplinary approach to the care of the STEMI patients throughout their entire journey. There is a demonstrated value in developing a sophisticated interprofessional STEMI system of care that begins with the EMS teams working in concert with ED staff and cardiology experts. This envisioned integrated system will best serve to prescreen, identify, consult, and implement an evidence-based therapy suited for the individual STEMI patient regardless of their location, age, or first point of medical contact. As Canada moves toward this envisioned system, we must continue to fortify and sophisticate our existing clinical systems while keeping a keen focus on research that will allow us to pave the best possible path for STEMI care into the future.

REFERENCES

1. Canadian Institute of Health Information 2010–2011. Available at: http://www.cihi.ca/CIHI-ext-portal/internet/EN/Home/home/cihi000001.
2. Patel AB, Tu JV, Waters NM, et al. Access to primary percutaneous coronary intervention for ST-segment elevation myocardial infarction in Canada: a geographic analysis. *Open Med.* 2010;4(1):e13–e21.
3. Schull MJ, Vaillancourt S, Donovan L, et al. Underuse of prehospital strategies to reduce time to reperfusion for ST-elevation myocardial infarction patients in 5 Canadian provinces. *Can J Emerg Med.* 2009;11(5):473–480.
4. Le May MR, So DY, Dionne R, et al. A citywide protocol for primary PCI in ST-segment elevation myocardial infarction. *N Engl J Med.* 2008;358(3):231–240.
5. de Villiers JS, Anderson T, McMeekin JD, et al. Expedited transfer for primary percutaneous coronary intervention: a program evaluation. *Can Med Assoc J.* 2007;176(13):1833–1838.
6. Ducas RA, Philipp RK, Jassal DS, et al. Cardiac Outcomes Through Digital Evaluation (CODE) STEMI project: prehospital digitally-assisted reperfusion strategies. *Can J Cardiol.* 2012;28(4):423–431.
7. Welsh RC. Computer-assisted paramedic electrocardiogram interpretation with remote physician over-read: the future of prehospital STEMI care? *Can J Cardiol.* 2012;28(4):408–410.
8. Welsh RC, Travers A, Senaratne M, Williams R, Armstrong PW. Feasibility and applicability of paramedic-based prehospital fibrinolysis in a large North American center. *Am Heart J.* 2006;152(6):1007–1014.
9. Welsh RC, Chang W, Goldstein P, et al. Time to treatment and the impact of a physician on prehospital management of acute ST elevation myocardial infarction: insights from the ASSENT-3 PLUS trial. *Heart.* 2005;91(11):1400–1406.
10. Armstrong PW, Gershlick AH, Goldstein P, et al. Fibrinolysis or primary PCI in ST-segment elevation myocardial infarction. *N Engl J Med.* 2013;368(15):1379–1387.
11. Shavadia J, Ibrahim Q, Sookram S, et al. Bridging the gap for non-metropolitan STEMI patients through implementation of a pharmacoinvasive reperfusion strategy. *Can J Cardiol.* 2013;29(8):951–959.

CHAPTER 9

Denmark: Prehospital STEMI Management Systems

Maria Sejersten, MD, DMSc, and
Peter Clemmensen, MD, DMSc

A NATIONAL TREATMENT STRATEGY FOR ACUTE MYOCARDIAL INFARCTION (AMI) PATIENTS

Ischemic heart disease is a leading course of death and disability in Denmark and causes more than 46,000 admissions every year. Nearly 16,000 of these are diagnosed with coronary artery disease, and 9000 with a myocardial infarction (MI).[1] Among patients with MI, 1 to 3 have electrocardiographic (ECG) changes meeting the criteria for ST-elevation myocardial infarction (STEMI),[2] and 2 to 3 are diagnosed with non-STEMI (NSTEMI).[3]

In 2003, as a result of the Danish trial in acute myocardial infarction-2 (DANAMI-2), the national strategy for treatment of STEMI in Denmark changed overnight from thrombolysis to primary percutaneous coronary intervention (PPCI).[4] This change was possible because during the course of the conduct of DANAMI-2, PPCI had already been established in five PPCI centers operating 24/7, with a large patient uptake, highly

Prehospital Management of Acute STEMI: Practical Approaches and International Strategies for Early Intervention © 2015 Joseph S. Alpert, Lynne T. Braun, Barbara J. Fletcher, Gerald Fletcher, Editors-in-Chief, Cardiotext Publishing, ISBN: 978-1-935395-66-9

experienced operators, and on-site cardiac surgery. Currently, four centers perform PPCI in Denmark, and 5 hospitals perform elective coronary angiography (CAG), with an additional three centers performing both CAG and elective PCI (Figure 9.1).

A well-functioning ambulance service, prehospital ECG recording and transmission, prehospital triage, and the widespread access to PPCI allows 70% to 80% of the Danish STEMI patients to be transferred directly to a PPCI center, bypassing local hospitals. The majority of these

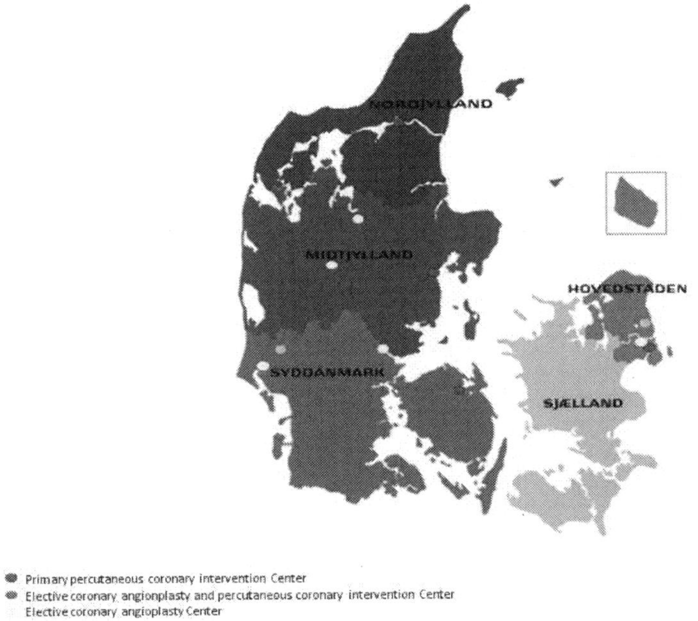

Figure 9.1

Denmark divided into the 5 healthcare regions (Hovedstaden, Sjælland, Syddanmark, Midtjylland, and Nordjylland), and the locations of the 4 centers performing primary percutaneous coronary intervention (PPCI), and the hospitals performing CAG, and elective PCI.

patients are treated within 120 minutes from first medical contact,[5,6] whereas patients with NSTEMI are offered CAG/PCI within 72 hours.[7] However, this achievement relies on several factors including infrastructure, logistics, and close cooperation among the interdisciplinary healthcare teams.

DEMOGRAPHICS AND THE PREHOSPITAL STRATEGY

Denmark is a fairly small country with 5.6 million inhabitants living in an area of 43,000 km^2, counting 406 islands of varying size, of which 71 are inhabited. Denmark is divided into five healthcare regions, each responsible for all prehospital and hospital treatments in the region. Eight emergency medical services (EMS) centers are distributed throughout the regions. They receive all 112 (911) calls and are responsible for dispatching the ambulances. Seven of the EMS centers are run by the police, and one is run by one of the regions.

The size of the country may case some challenges in ensuring early and uniform prehospital treatment to all, but historically an overall prehospital contingency plan has not been available until recently. The Danish Healthcare Quality Program (DDKM) is an accreditation system, and the program serves as a method to generate continuous and persistent quality development across the entire healthcare sector in Denmark.[8] The DDKM provides accreditation standards of good quality, along with methods to measure and control this quality. Because the first version of the DDKM program for the prehospital setting was issued in 2011, prehospital treatment is still not completely standardized throughout the country and treatment may still vary according to area, distance to a major city, and time of the day.

INVOLVING THE GENERAL PUBLIC IN THE STEMI MANAGEMENT TEAM THROUGH CARDIOPULMONARY RESUSCITATION (CPR) TRAINING

STEMI patients are in danger of experiencing cardiac arrest during the first hours of symptom onset, typically by malignant ventricular arrhythmias or cardiogenic shock. Up to 10% experience cardiac arrest and die before hospital arrival.[9] The number of Danes capable of initiating basic resuscitation continues to increase, because everyone must pass a course of basic resuscitation to obtain a Danish drivers license. General knowledge of basic resuscitation has increased the chance of surviving cardiac arrest outside a hospital,[10] and the chance of surviving is also increasing with the general availability of automated external defibrillators (AEDs).[11]

Over the years, approximately 15,000 AEDs have been purchased and installed in both private and public locations, indoors and outside, all over Denmark (Table 9.1). To ensure quality and effort, the Danish Health and Medicines Authority has issued common standards for registration, installation, education, quality control, monitoring, and the purchase of AEDs.[12] By May 2014, the location of 9878 AEDs were registered on the website www.hjertestarter.dk. All healthcare personnel answering 112 calls at the EMS centers have passed a course on cardiac resuscitation using an AED and can assist the caller accordingly. They can also direct the caller to the nearest AED location using data from the www.hjertestarter.dk website. To ensure proper service of the device, the cardiac resuscitation network is alerted when an AED has been used.

Table 9.1
Placement of automatic external defibrillators in Denmark

	Percent (%)
Businesses (accountant, factory, etc.)	26.8
Sport grounds	18.4
State/local authority	9.9
School/university	9.6
General physician, dentist, health center, and so forth	6.8
Institution (daycare, nursery home, etc.)	4.5
Culture (museum, theatre, library, church, etc.)	4.1
Other (harbor, ferry, airport, private home, etc.)	7.7

SHORTENING PREHOSPITAL DELAYS TO EMS ARRIVAL

There has been no recent national campaign in Denmark to inform the general population to seek medical treatment acutely in cases of chest pain. However, the Danish Heart Foundation plays an important part in providing continual general information about heart disease, and in addition, the major news effect after the DANAM-2 trial[4] may have increased the awareness of ischemic heart disease in Denmark. Patient delay (time from symptom onset to 112 call) is related to the acuteness of the patients symptoms, and is longer in patients with uncharacteristic versus classic symptoms. Two Danish studies have reported fairly short patient delays of 37 to 60 minutes.[13,14]

The Danish government urges EMS help to be provided within 15 minutes under normal circumstances, but each region decides what time frame to pursue. Generally, the goal is that 75% of the ambulances arrive within 10 minutes of the 112 call. In an urban area, a dispatch time (time from

112 call to ambulance arrival) of 6 minutes has been reported in a study of patients with chest pain,[14] but longer times are expected in rural areas (Table 9.2). In the same Danish study, scene time increased by 7 minutes after the implementation of ECG recording and ECG transmission from the ambulance. However, the increased time was compensated by early notice and assembly of the catheterization team at the PPCI centers prior to patient arrival.

AMBULANCE SERVICE UNIFORMITY IN DENMARK

Denmark is unique because one ambulance service (Falck) covers the vast majority (~85%) of the country, and 4 other ambulance services cover the remainder. The first advantage is uniform prehospital care and treatment. Second, because the majority of the ambulances in Denmark carry the same equipment for ECG recording and transmission (Lifepak 15, Physio-Control, Inc., Redmond, WA), technology needs are simplified by not requiring several systems to interact; for example, the hospitals only need one receiving station for receiving transmitted ECGs.

The primary ambulance is staffed with emergency medical technicians (EMTs) and in some cases a paramedic. The EMT can defibrillate when needed, and administer oral aspirin, oral nitroglycerin, and oxygen. Paramedics are educated in administrating intravenous medication and will, in addition to defibrillation, be able to treat the most common arrhythmic complications by intravenous medication. Transport times differ according to the distance between the patient and the PPCI center. The longest transport distances in Denmark are nearly 200 km, and transport times up to 3 hours can be expected.

An advanced emergency medical unit (AMU) manned with a paramedic and/or a physician provides support to the

Table 9.2
Prehospital ambulance service in the 5 regions in Denmark

	Region Hovedstaden	Region Sjælland	Region Syddanmark	Region Midtjylland	Region Nordjylland
Ambulance operator	FALCK Copenhagen fire department Frederiksberg fire department	FALCK Roskilde fire department	FALCK	FALCK Respons Samsø redningskorps	FALCK
Model	Contingency	Response time	Response time	Contingency	Response time
Response time (minutes)	50% within 6.5 90% within 13	8.1–9.5	50% with 6.7 90% within 13	75% with 10 92% within 15 98% within 20 Mean 7.5	95% within 20 Mean 9.12
Number of ambulances	47	50	56	64	54

(*Continued*)

Table 9.2
(Continued)

	Region Hovedstaden	Region Sjælland	Region Syddanmark	Region Midtjylland	Region Nordjylland
Number of emergency medical units per million people	1.88	2	3.75	2.44	1.63
Number of emergency medical units per 10,000 km^2	12	2.24	3.66	2.28	1.19
Emergency medical units manned by	Anesthesiologist + paramedic	Paramedic	Anesthesiologist, or general practitioner or paramedic	Anesthesiologist, or general practitioner, or paramedic	Anesthesiologist + paramedic, or military-trained MD

Contingency model: the region dictates the number of ambulances. Response time model: the ambulance operator dictates the number of ambulances.
(Data from Kindberg et al., *Ugeskr laeger.* 2009;171:2553–2557.)

primary ambulance, depending on the local regions' prehospital service.[15] The AMU is dispatched simultaneously and rendezvous with the primary ambulance to the site of 112 call or en route to the hospital. The AMU can initiate advanced treatments but cannot transport patients, which is carried out by the primary ambulance.

PREHOSPITAL ECG RECORDING AND TRANSMISSION REQUIRED BY LAW

Prehospital 12-lead ECG acquisition and transmission is now the standard of care, as required by law, in Denmark.[16,17] One of the first national initiatives to improve prehospital care, including up-stream diagnosis and treatment in cardiac patients, was a healthcare departmental bill from 2000 ordering all ambulances in Denmark to be equipped with defibrillators and a device for 12-lead ECG recording and transmission.[17] By 2008, all ambulances in Denmark carried such a device. Continuing education in 12-lead ECG acquisition, transmission, and interpretation as well as cardiac pathophysiology are integral parts of the training program for ambulance personnel.[16,17] Consequently, all patients suspicious of acute coronary syndrome will have an ECG recorded and transmitted to the nearest PPCI center. This technology allows remote diagnosis and facilitates triage of STEMI patients to reperfusion therapy, and the initiation of adjunctive therapies within the prehospital setting. In addition, the receiving hospital obtains early notification of incoming patients and can prepare for appropriate treatment and activation of the catheterization laboratory when needed.[14,18]

The 12-lead ECG is transmitted from the ambulance via the global system for mobile communication (GSM) network to a receiving station located in the cardiac care unit at one of the four PPCI centers, where it is stored, displayed, and printed. Simultaneously, the ECG can be forwarded to the attending cardiologist's mobile phone or personal digital assistant. In addition, a web-based catalog of the latest 20 transmitted ECGs can be viewed on any hospital computer (Figure 9.2).

Continuous 12-lead ECG is established in all chest pain patients during transport to the hospital, in addition to monitoring arterial oxygen saturation and blood pressure. The ECG machines/defibrillators have algorithms for continuous monitoring of the ST segment. An alarm will sound or a new 12-lead ECG will be recorded in cases of ST-segment baseline changes beyond a certain threshold for a given amount of time. This allows the ambulance personnel to identify and react to changes in the ST segment indicating myocardial ischemia or infarction.

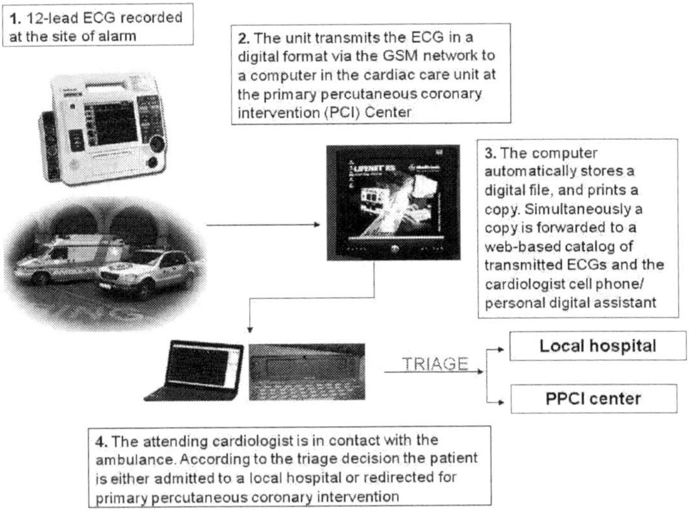

Figure 9.2

ECG transmission setup.

Both ST-segment monitoring and ECG diagnosis rely on the quality of the equipment as well as accurate electrode placement. However, placement of the precordial electrodes in their correct positions according to skeletal landmarks identified by palpation is challenging and time consuming, even for skilled personnel. Thus, ambulance personnel are continuously educated in the correct procedures for recording and transmitting the 12-lead ECG. Precordial electrodes are placed in the standard positions as accurately as possible, whereas limb electrodes are placed according to the Mason-Likar positions on the torso.[19]

PREHOSPITAL TRIAGE BY CARDIOLOGY FELLOWS AND INTERVENTIONAL CARDIOLOGISTS

Although the ambulance personnel are educated in recording and transmitting ECGs, the final diagnosis and triage decision rest upon the attending cardiologist fellow who is on-call 24/7 at one of the four centers performing PPCI in Denmark. In cases of uncertainty of the STEMI diagnosis, the fellow can contact the interventional cardiologist or attending cardiologist for a consult. The great advantage of this setup is the direct contact between the ambulance and a cardiology specialist with decision-making competence and the ability to activate the catheterization laboratory. With the cardiologist's experience, it may also be possible to reduce the number of times the catheterization laboratory is activated because of an incorrect diagnosis.

In some cases, remote contact between the cardiology fellow at the call center and the patient in transport is even possible. At one of the PPCI centers in Denmark (Skejby University Hospital), the cardiologist fellow is not only in contact with the ambulance personnel, but via a head-set in direct contact with the patient. By this setup, the cardiologist fellow can interview the patient and obtain valuable information needed for the triage decision. No study has compared the approach of triage decision with or without patient contact, but both setups have shown a significant reduction in time to PPCI,[14,18] while ECG transmission in general has been associated with lower mortality.[20]

Approximately 20,000 prehospital ECGs are transmitted from the ambulances to the four PPCI centers on a yearly basis (personal communication). Real-life triage in a Danish study of chest pain patients based on prehospital ECG transmission showed that 87% of patients referred for PPCI received immediate catherization (PPCI in 80%, CAG only in 19%, and emergent bypass surgery in 1%).[14] Of patients not receiving an intervention, half died before PPCI could be initiated or declined invasive treatment, and the other half were reevaluated upon hospital arrival and had no indication for PPCI.[14] STEMI was confirmed in 79% of patients referred directly for PPCI. Only 6% of patients admitted at local hospitals after the on-call cardiologist fellow had judged them not to have STEMI were diagnosed with STEMI at hospital discharge. Another Danish study showed that 70% of all STEMI patients are field-triaged directly to a PPCI centers on the basis of prehospital ECG transmission. The remaining STEMI patients are walk-ins or patients without diagnostic ECG changes initially triaged to the local hospital emergency department or trauma center.[21]

Walk-in patients and patients initially triaged to a local hospital are transferred to the PPCI center either by an ambulance or a helicopter depending on the distance between the local referring hospital and the PPCI center. Helicopters are most often used if the distance is beyond 90 km. Occasionally, the same primary ambulance can be used in case of new ECG developments en route or immediately upon arrival to the local hospital. Otherwise a new ambulance is requested. The major challenge in timely treatment in this group of STEMI patients is not the availability of ambulance transfer, but rather the procedures associated with consulting and patient-related preparation, which causes long door-in, door-out times up to 60 minutes.[4]

PREHOSPITAL ANTITHROMBOTIC THERAPY AND TRANSPORTATION PROTOCOLS IN DENMARK

All acute coronary syndrome patients receive dual-antiplatelet therapy with oral aspirin (300 mg loading dose) and either prasugrel (60 mg loading dose), ticagrelor (180 mg loading dose), or clopidogrel (600 mg loading dose). Anticoagulation with intravenous unfractionated heparin is administered to STEMI patients after the diagnosis is confirmed by transmission of the ECG to the on-call cardiologist fellow.

Complications are expected in the early hours after manifestation of STEMI, and consequently safe ambulance transport is pivotal. The Danish Society of Cardiology recommends rendezvous by an AMU (preferably with a physician) in all transports of unstable STEMI patients (persistent arrhythmia, need for intubation, or cardiogenic shock) and rendezvous if possible when transporting stable STEMI patients.[22]

EXPANDED HELICOPTER SERVICE

The Danish hospital setting is undergoing reorganization, with smaller hospitals closing and large hospitals/emergency departments evolving, and thus distances between patients and hospitals are increasing. One possible solution is the use of helicopters to ensure that patients living far from the nearest hospital are offered equally good prehospital help and expedient transport to a hospital in cases of severe illness or emergencies. A helicopter service operated with MBB/Kawasaki BK 117 helicopters was introduced during daytime flight hours in 2010 in the eastern part of Denmark (Zealand). The following year, a similar service was introduced in the western part of Denmark (Jutland), but with the helicopter operating 24/7 and capable of flying in the dark. Standard interdisciplinary personnel on these helicopters are an experienced physician (a specialist in anesthesiology and trained in emergency medicine), a pilot, and a paramedic.

A recent study showed that patients with a transport distance of more than 60 km to the PPCI center may benefit from helicopter transportation, and that transportation by helicopter was associated with a delay of less than 120 minutes even at a transport distance up to 150 km. Surprisingly, patients living up to 150 km from a PPCI center were treated with PPCI only 30 minutes later than patients living close by a PPCI center.[23] The study showed the importance of correct placement of helicopter bases in remote areas closest to the patients with the largest benefit potential to optimize response time and operation radius. Preferably, the primary ambulance and helicopter are dispatched simultaneously. It is recommended that the helicopters be able to operate at night and in poor visibility, and be manned by a physician experienced in emergency medicine. Communication between the helicopter and the receiving department is pivotal, as well as the ability of the helicopter to operate directly between patient pickup and hospital without the involvement of an ambulance. The helicopter service became nationwide in Denmark in 2013.

In addition, an airborne search and rescue (SAR) service operated by the Danish Air service has been integrated into the prehospital STEMI system such that patients from the remote island Bornholm in the Baltic Sea have been transferred for PPCI since 2005. In this setting, after the patient calls 112 and primary ambulance dispatch, the ambulance personnel alerts the attending cardiologist at the island hospital in case of a tentative STEMI diagnosis. Then the attending cardiologist fellow at nearest PPCI center is notified and activates the air force transfer. SAR transfer of STEMI patients is performed with an AgustaWestland EH101 Merlin helicopter, and one-way flight time from Bornholm to the nearest PPCI center is currently 45 minutes. Roof-top helipads at the PPCI center and a dedicated helipad adjacent to the emergency department at the island hospital have been installed to save valuable time.

CONCLUSION

In Denmark, close collaboration and communication among interdisciplinary teams within EMS, local hospitals, PPCI centers, and a private or military helicopter ambulance service ensures a well-organized STEMI network. Legislation has helped to mandate key parts of prehospital program implementation, such as CPR training among the public who obtain driver's licenses and a standard of care for prehospital 12-lead ECG acquisition and transmission by EMS. Because the majority of the ambulances in Denmark carry the same equipment for ECG recording and transmission, some of the logistical difficulties of coordinating these efforts have been reduced. Field triage of STEMI uses call centers staffed by cardiology fellows. These highly integrated systems and the widespread access to PPCI in Denmark have produced a prehospital STEMI management system where most patients can be treated within the time limits suggested by the current guidelines. This overall organization of prehospital care is likely to contribute to the reduced mortality rate of STEMI patients in Denmark.

REFERENCES

1. Nissen NK, Rasmussen S. *Hjertestatistik 2008*. Copenhagen: Hjerteforeningen i samarbejde med Statens Institut for Folkesundhed, Syddansk Universitet, 2008.

2. Thygesen K, Alpert JS, White HD, et al. Universal definition of myocardial infarction. *Circulation.* 2007;116:2634–2653.
3. Jensen LO, Thayssen P. [Treatment and prognosis after acute coronary syndrome in an unselected patient population]. *Ugeskr Laeger.* 2007;169:492–497.
4. Andersen HR, Nielsen TT, Rasmussen K, et al. A comparison of coronary angioplasty with fibrinolytic therapy in acute myocardial infarction. *N Engl J Med.* 2003;349:733–742.
5. Schoos MM, Sejersten M, Hvelplund A, et al. Reperfusion delay in patients treated with primary percutaneous coronary intervention: insight from a real world Danish ST-segment elevation myocardial infarction population in the era of telemedicine. *Eur Heart J: Acute Cardiovasc Care.* 2012;1:200–209.
6. Sorensen JT, Terkelsen CJ, Norgaard BL, et al. Urban and rural implementation of pre-hospital diagnosis and direct referral for primary percutaneous coronary intervention in patients with acute ST-elevation myocardial infarction. *Eur Heart J.* 2011;32:430–436.
7. Sundhedsstyrelsen. Pakkeforløb for UAP og NSTEMI. 1.1. 1 October 2009.
8. Hundborg K. [The Danish Quality Model]. *Ugeskr Laeger.* 2009;171:1660–1663.
9. Gheeraert PJ, De Buyzere ML, Taeymans YM, et al. Risk factors for primary ventricular fibrillation during acute myocardial infarction: a systematic review and meta-analysis. *Eur Heart J.* 2006;27:2499–2510.
10. Rea TD, Eisenberg MS, Culley LL, Becker L. Dispatcher-assisted cardiopulmonary resuscitation and survival in cardiac arrest. *Circulation.* 2001;104:2513–2516.
11. Nielsen AM, Folke F, Lippert FK, Rasmussen LS. Use and benefits of public access defibrillation in a nation-wide network. *Resuscitation.* 2013;84(4):430–434.
12. Sundshedsstyrrelsen. Hjertestartere (AED) placeret uden for sygehus. Sundhedsstyrrelsen. 1 November 2011.
13. Jensen J, Christensen PB. [Delays in admissions for observation in suspected acute myocardial infarction]. *Ugeskr Laeger.* 1993;155:2892–2896.
14. Sejersten M, Sillesen M, Hansen PR, et al. Effect on treatment delay of prehospital teletransmission of 12-lead electrocardiogram to a cardiologist for immediate triage and direct referral of patients with ST-segment elevation acute myocardial infarction to primary percutaneous coronary intervention. *Am J Cardiol.* 2008;101:941–946.
15. Kindberg K, Nielsen SL, Møller AM. Præhospitale lægebaserede behandlinger i Danmark. *Ugeskr Laeger.* 2009;171:2553–2557.
16. Bekendtgørelse om planlægning af sundhedsberedskabet og det præhospitale beredskab samt uddannelse af ambulancepersonale m.v. nr 977. 26 September 2006.

17. Bekendtgørelse nr. 1039 af 24/11/2000 om planlægning af den præhospitale indsats og uddannelse af ambulancepersonale m.v. 1039. 2000.
18. Terkelsen CJ, Lassen JF, Norgaard BL, et al. Reduction of treatment delay in patients with ST-elevation myocardial infarction: impact of pre-hospital diagnosis and direct referral to primary percutanous coronary intervention. *Eur Heart J.* 2005;26:770–777.
19. Mason RE, Likar I. A new system of multiple-lead exercise electrocardiography. *Am Heart J.* 1966;71:196–205.
20. Pedersen SH, Galatius S, Hansen PR, et al. Field triage reduces treatment delay and improves long-term clinical outcome in patients with acute ST-segment elevation myocardial infarction treated with primary percutaneous coronary intervention. *J Am Coll Cardiol.* 2009;54:2296–2302.
21. Terkelsen CJ, Jensen LO, Tilsted HH, et al. Primary percutaneous coronary intervention as a national reperfusion strategy in patients with ST-segment elevation myocardial infarction. *Circ Cardiovasc Interv.* 2011;4:570–576.
22. Niemann T, Holmvang L. Den Nationale kardiologiske Behandlingsvejledning - NBV2009. Præ- og interhospitaltransport af hjertepatienter. 2009.
23. Knudsen L, Stengaard C, Hansen TM, Lassen JF, Terkelsen CJ. Earlier reperfusion in patients with ST-elevation myocardial infarction by use of helicopter. *Scand J Trauma Resusc Emerg Med.* 2012;20:70.

CHAPTER 10

Argentina: Prehospital Management of STEMI

Liliana Grinfeld, PhD, and Florencia Rolandi, MD, MSc

ARGENTINA: DEMOGRAPHICS AND HEALTHCARE SYSTEM RESOURCES

Acute myocardial infarction and its related complications continue to be among the highest-risk events for coronary artery disease patients. Sudden cardiac death in the very early stage is still a very difficult problem to solve. Patients with ST-elevation myocardial infarction (STEMI) who reach medical assistance should be managed according to the standard of care of the region, taking into consideration that even within the same region, there are different approaches depending on each hospital's facilities.

The present situation in Argentina shows educational, social, economic, and medical coverage inequalities that make access to evidence-based therapies disparate across the entire population.

According to estimates from the National Institute of Statistics and Census (INDEC), in Argentina there were 40,518,951 inhabitants in 2010, most living in urban areas.[1] Life expectancy at birth is 75.2 years overall: 79.1 years for women and 71.6 years for men. Health provision is covered by 3 sectors: public, private, and medical insurance, but nearly 36% of the population does not have any health coverage. Updated data indicate that public spending on health represents 6.21% of the gross domestic product (GDP) and

Prehospital Management of Acute STEMI: Practical Approaches and International Strategies for Early Intervention © 2015 Joseph S. Alpert, Lynne T. Braun, Barbara J. Fletcher, Gerald Fletcher, Editors-in-Chief, Cardiotext Publishing, ISBN: 978-1-935395-66-9

almost half of the inpatient care facilities belong to the public sector.

ESTIMATIONS OF INCIDENCE AND MORTALITY OF MYOCARDIAL INFARCTION IN ARGENTINA

In Argentina, cardiovascular disease is responsible for about one-third of deaths in both men and women. Cardiovascular mortality showed an increase in recent years. The crude and adjusted cardiovascular death rates were, respectively, 227.33 and 199.15 per 100,000 inhabitants in 2008 versus 239.44 and 204.00 per 100,000 inhabitants in 2010.[1,2]

No population-based statistics allow us to know the exact incidence of acute myocardial infarction. However, analysis based on data from small towns, as well as many surveys, suggest that at least 35,000 patients suffer an acute myocardial infarction each year.[3,4] In terms of prognosis, periodic reports have been published by the scientific societies in the last 20 years showing information on hospital mortality.[5-10] But although these surveys represent an important effort from the researchers, most of them have significant methodological limitations such as selection bias when including referral hospitals, the small sample size analyzed, and the lack of monitoring and quality control of data (Figure 10.1).

LOCAL THERAPEUTIC STRATEGIES

Recent surveys show that over 40% of patients with STEMI in Argentina do not receive any therapy (Figure 10.2). Assuming the estimate of approximately 35,000 infarctions per year, the amount of nonreperfused patients may be higher than reported. In fact, in 2008 the Argentine College of Interventional Cardioangiologists (CACI) reported that nearly

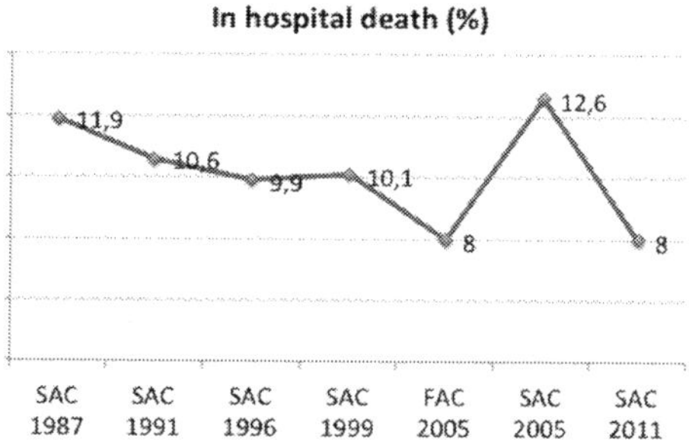

Figure 10.1

In-hospital death according to surveys. Data labeled "SAC" + date indicate the Argentine Cardiology Society surveys during different periods of time.

3500 percutaneous coronary interventions (PCIs) were performed in patients reported with acute myocardial infarction. On the other hand, the leading provider of streptokinase, the locally most frequently used thrombolytic, estimated annual sales of 4600 doses. One of the main reasons for nonuse of reperfusion therapy has been attributed to late hospital arrival, outside the time of the therapeutic window. Other mentioned

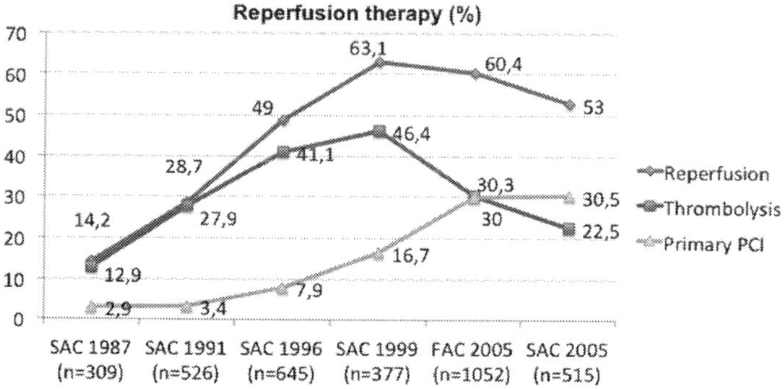

Figure 10.2

Reperfusion strategies. Data are from Argentine Cardiology Society (SAC) and Argentine Cardiology Federation's surveys during different periods of time.[5-10]

causes are older age and lack of availability of thrombolytics, both of which are modifiable with medical education and adequate provision of resources.

COMPONENTS OF PREHOSPITAL STEMI MANAGEMENT IN ARGENTINA

Most patients with STEMI are treated with thrombolytics, though the number of primary percutaneous coronary intervention (PPCI) performed yearly is increasing, especially in the private sectors. Management of patients in the public sector is not standardized. Even in Buenos Aires, the largest city of Argentina, there are relatively few public hospitals with 24-hour PPCI capabilities.

Buenos Aires boasts 3 million inhabitants, but on weekdays during working hours, the number jumps to 10 million. The city has 15 public hospitals, of which three have catheterization labs available only during working hours on weekdays, and only three have 24/7 PPCI facilities. Emergency calls are centralized in a 911 phone number. Patients are transferred by ambulances that are equipped with monitors and defibrillators, but without ECG machines, to the nearest site. Patients are treated according to each hospital's standard of care. At hospitals without a cath lab, they are usually treated with thrombolytics, and some hospitals routinely transfer patients for angioplasty after the thrombolysis, adopting a pharmacoinvasive approach. However, a new program for transferring patients for PPCI has been proposed by the Health Ministry of Buenos Aires. This program should guarantee the transfer of patients from sites without PPCI facilities to an available cath lab in less than 60 minutes.

There is still no formal national strategy for prehospital thrombolytic administration in Argentina; therefore, according to the latest guidelines presented by the Argentine Cardiology Society (SAC), prehospital thrombolysis with the use of a bolus fibrinolytic is included as a class I indication, if a primary angioplasty cannot be performed in less than 90 minutes in high-risk infarcts.[11] This is a very attractive idea, considering the geographical features of Argentina with long distances between towns and heavy traffic in the cities. Argentina is somewhat different from many other countries in that ambulances are actually staffed by a physician. This offers additional options for the ambulance physician to send and interpret the ECG and assess the clinical condition of the patient.

RECOMMENDATIONS FOR IMPROVEMENT

Public Awareness and Education

Public awareness and education is one of the key starting points. The general population usually has very little information regarding symptoms that could be related to acute myocardial infarction other than severe chest pain. A survey performed by SAC and its foundation evaluated the level of awareness and knowledge about symptoms and coronary risk factors. The results showed that people learned more about cardiovascular diseases from the media than from their physicians.[12] With these observations, the foundation developed several TV and radio campaigns instructing the population to identify signs and symptoms that could be related to heart attacks and to seek medical assistance.

Prevention

Scientific societies, foundations, and public health authorities in Argentina have all been involved in promoting prevention of heart disease. These efforts include several programs alerting the public about cardiovascular risk factors, opening public centers for those seeking help with smoking cessation, and providing obesity treatment and counseling. In addition, educational programs for children and adolescents have been launched, teaching them healthy habits. The good part of this public awareness is that most of the programs are free of charge, and there is a lot of information easily available. Unfortunately, there is no coordination among all these efforts.

Policies and Standard Recommendations for Management of STEMI Patients

All scientific societies related to the management of acute myocardial infarction patients have agreed to a common set of recommendations, drafting a document that proposes the development of active policies by the same scientific societies and health authorities.[13] The objective is to adopt a basic standard for acute myocardial infarction assistance at different stages, through implementation of educational interventions to the general community and health professionals, the provision of adequate resources in all segments of the healthcare system, and the record of quality measurement tools for an ongoing evaluation of the effectiveness of the actions taken.

The report considers that, given the heterogeneity of the system of health care by geographical area and coverage, it is imperative to develop a series of steps to configure a quality standard of prehospital and in-hospital management of patients with acute myocardial infarction, which can be evaluated and improved in performance. Basically, it should ensure the following: rapid implementation and interpretation of the ECG in the prehospital phase, early reperfusion with thrombolytics or angioplasty, and regionalization of care, structuring a network for referral of critically ill patients. The latter is in line with international guidelines that recommended as class I indication the creation of a regional network of hospitals of varying complexity.[14]

Specifically in the prehospital phase, the quality standard, as a suggestion, should ensure that ambulances are equipped with ECG and defibrillator, as well as a system for transmitting the results to a central system with highly trained operators. In Argentina, the ambulances have a physician, so it should be easier to implement training for staff who have the first medical contact with the patient not only to make the correct diagnosis, but also to initiate treatment through the use of thrombolytics, ideally in bolus form. Educating the population to seek medical care early, ensuring the provision of inputs and trained human resources and, fundamentally, the articulated work between scientific societies, healthcare institutions and health authorities, can turn the prehospital thrombolysis theory into practice.

CONCLUSION

Cardiovascular mortality has continued to show an increase in recent years in Argentina, and most patients with STEMI are treated with thrombolytics, though the number of PPCI performed yearly is increasing, especially in the private sectors.

Scientific societies, foundations, and public health authorities in Argentina have all been involved in promoting prevention of heart disease and providing recommendations for a quality standard of prehospital and in-hospital management of patients with acute myocardial infarction, which can be evaluated and improved in performance. The heterogeneity of the system of health care by geographical area and available services make it imperative to develop a series of steps to configure a quality standard of care.

REFERENCES

1. Ministerio de Salud de la Nación, Dirección de Estadísticas e Información de Salud. Serie 5 No 54, "Estadísticas Vitales. Información Básica 2010". Buenos Aires, Argentina, 2011.
2. Ministerio de Salud de la Nación. Dirección de Estadísticas e Información de Salud. Serie 5 No 52/09 "Estadísticas Vitales. Información Básica 2008". Buenos Aires, Argentina, 2009.
3. Caccavo A, Alvarez A, Bello FH, et al. Incidencia poblacional del infarto con elevación del STo bloqueo de rama izquierda a lo largo de 11 años en una comunidad de la provincia de Buenos Aires. *Rev Argent Cardiol.* 2007;75:185–188.
4. Ferrante D, Tajer CD. ¿Cuántos infartos hay en la Argentina? *Rev Argent Cardiol.* 2007;75:161–162.
5. Gagliardi J, Lipschitz S, Cecchi A, Shifres A, Tajer C. Consejo de Emergencias SAC - CONAREC. Infarto Agudo de Miocardio en la Capital Federal. Registro Prospectivo. Congreso Internacional 50o Aniversario de la Sociedad Argentina de Cardiología. Abstract. *Rev Argent Cardiol.* 1987;55:4.
6. Sociedad Argentina de Cardiología. Encuesta Nacional de Unidades Coronarias. *Rev Argent Cardiol.* 1991;59(suppl 2):7–40.
7. Hirschson Prado A, Trivi M, Tajer C, Charask A, et al. Infarto agudo de miocardio en la Argentina. Tercera Encuesta Nacional SAC 1996. *Rev Argent Cardiol.* 1998;66(1):63–72.
8. Kevorkian R, Blanco P, Ferreirós E, Higa C, et al. en representación de los investigadores del Registro IAM-1999, de los miembros del Área de Investigación de la Sociedad Argentina de Cardiología y de la Sociedad Argentina de Cardiología. Registro IAM- 1999. *Rev Argent Cardiol.* 2001;69:488–500.
9. Zapata G. Registro Nacional de Infarto Agudo de Miocardio de la Federación Argentina de Cardiología. Etapa III. *Rev Fed Arg Cardiol.* 2006;35:130–132.
10. Blanco P, Gagliardi J, Higa C, et al. Infarto agudo de miocardio. Resultados de la Encuesta SAC 2005 en la República Argentina. *Rev Argent Cardiol.* 2007;75:163–170.
11. Pomés Iparraguirre H, Consenso SCA con supradesnivel del ST. XXXV Congreso Argentino de Cardiología. Buenos Aires, 3 de octubre de, 2009.
12. Rolandi F, Grinfeld L, Sosa Liprandi MI, et al. Encuesta de reconocimiento de la enfermedad cardiovascular en la mujer por la mujer. *Rev Argent Cardiol.* 2013;81:308–314.
13. Documento de la Sociedad Argentina de Cardiología (SAC), la Federación Argentina de Cardiología (FAC), la Sociedad Argentina de Terapia Intensiva (SATI), el Colegio Argentino de Cardioangiólogos Intervencionistas (CACI), la Fundación

Cardiológica Argentina (FCA), la Sociedad Argentina de Patología de Urgencia y Emergentología (SAPUE) y el Consejo Argentino de Residentes de Cardiología (CONAREC). Realidad del manejo del infarto agudo de miocardio con elevación del segmento ST en la Argentina. *Rev Argent Cardiol.* 2008;76:226–228.

14. O'Gara PT, Kushner FG, Ascheim DD, et al. 2013 ACCF/AHA guideline for the management of ST-elevation myocardial infarction: a report of the American College of Cardiology Foundation/American Heart Association Task Force on Practice Guidelines. *Circulation.* 2013;127:e362–e425.

CHAPTER 11

Brazil: Prehospital Management of STEMI

Roberto Vieira Botelho, MD, PhD, and Thais Waisman, MD, PhD

DEMOGRAPHICS AND HEALTHCARE DELIVERY SYSTEMS IN BRAZIL

Worldwide, it is estimated that death from coronary heart disease (CHD) will increase 100% in men and 80% in women from 1990 to 2020, with the majority of that increase coming from Asia, Africa, and Latin America.[1] Similarly, disability-adjusted life-years lost will increase 107% in men and 74% in women worldwide.[1]

Brazil is a continental country of 8,514,876,599 km^2. Almost 75% of the population depends on the public unified health system (SUS). In 2000, the Brazilian population was 184 million people, distributed in 5564 cities that were supplied by 65,343 health facilities. Among them, 38,347 were public facilities, and only 2589 of these were able to hospitalize patients.[2,3]

Despite the superiority of primary percutaneous coronary intervention (PPCI) compared with thrombolysis for the treatment of acute myocardial infarction (AMI), only 330 catheterization labs are available across the country, most of which are concentrated in the big cities. Since 2004, the number of primary angioplasties has increased significantly, from 1901 patients in 2004, to 5400 patients in 2005, 6605 in 2006, 7551

Prehospital Management of Acute STEMI: Practical Approaches and International Strategies for Early Intervention © 2015 Joseph S. Alpert, Lynne T. Braun, Barbara J. Fletcher, Gerald Fletcher, Editors-in-Chief, Cardiotext Publishing, ISBN: 978-1-935395-66-9

in 2007, and 7648 in 2008.[4] Despite the significant growth, it is an unacceptably low utilization of this approach for the treatment of AMI.

The Brazilian distribution of physicians follows the per capita income (Table 11.1). The area of Brasilia (Federal District, DF), with an annual per capita income of approximately US$8000, has 3.42 physicians per thousand inhabitants; however, the state of Maranhão (MA), with an annual US$928 per capita income, has 0.56 physicians per thousand inhabitants.[5] The association of higher incidence of AMI, lower infrastructure, and lower number of physicians creates a critical paradox for the healthcare system. Those who need care the most, receive the least.

The Brazilian annual health budget is around US$80 billion, but the distribution is quite unequal. Half of the budget covers approximately 50 million people under the private/health insurance system, and the other US$40 billion inadequately covers the remaining 140 million people in the public system.[6]

Table 11.1
Brazilian physicians per 1000 inhabitants and per capita GDP

State	Per capita GDP	Physicians/1000 inhabitants
DF	R$16,361	3.42
RJ	R$11,459	3.35
SP	R$11,353	2.23
RS	R$9958	2.02
AP	R$4996	0.82
TO	R$2931	0.97
PI	R$2113	0.78
MA	R$1949	0.56

R, Brazilian Reais (unit of currency); GDP, gross domestic product; DF, Federal District; RJ, state of Rio de Janeiro; SP, state of São Paulo; RS, state of Rio Grande do Sul; AP, state of Amapa; TO, state of Tocantins; PI, state of Piaui; MA, state of Maranhão.

In an effort to overcome this challenging scenario, the Brazilian Ministry of Health has created a dedicated chapter for the diagnosis and treatment of acute coronary syndrome (ACS). Highlighted is the Mobile Urgency Service (SAMU) prepared for delivering thrombolytics in the field after the support of a telemedicine prehospital ECG.[7]

PARTICULAR CONSIDERATIONS FOR THE PREHOSPITAL SITUATION IN BRAZIL

Like many countries, Brazil has a specific geography and population distribution that are factors in prehospital ST-segment elevation myocardial infarction (STEMI) management.

The Economic Cost of Chest Pain Triage

The most frequent cause of emergency department visits is chest pain. It represents 10% of all cases, approximately 2,500,000 patients across the entire country every year. Among these patients, almost 70% do not have heart disease; however, they demand an enormous triage effort. Screening 30% of patients with threatening cardiovascular disease, mostly ACS, is the largest challenge for any health system, particularly in developing countries.[8] To hospitalize a chest pain patient may cost US$80,000 per quality-adjusted life-year.[9] The results are clear: overtriage, inappropriate triage that leads to excess hospitalization of "normal" patients, and undertriage, or inadequate treatment of acute cases.

Prehospital Delays

The factors related to prehospital delay are socioeconomic, clinical, environmental, cognitive, and emotional in nature.[10]

The Global Registry of Acute Coronary Events showed that patients from Brazil and Argentina had even greater prehospital delay compared with those from the United States and Canada.[11] The authors discussed that patient culture, lack of infrastructure, and logistics were mainly responsible for the difference.

Increasing Pprehospital Mortality for STEMI

There is a large difference between in-hospital and out-of-hospital mortality in Brazil. Out-of hospital mortality accounts for approximately two-thirds of all deaths from CHD,[12] whereas in the 1970s and early 1980s, in-hospital and out-of-hospital mortality fell in parallel fashion; more recent data from the late 1980s and 1990s found in-hospital mortality falling more rapidly. Sudden, out-of-hospital death comprises an increasing proportion of the mortality burden. Furthermore, these trends are not equally manifest in all ethnic groups, with the poor and ethnic minorities manifesting less positive changes.[13] Brazilian national data from DATASUS shows that 50% of AMI mortality will occur before hospital arrival and almost 60% of all MI deaths will occur in the first 2 hours of AMI onset.[14]

Despite strong evidence of its benefits, prehospital thrombolysis rates are still low. The challenge is to empower community practitioners to deliver thrombolysis. Telemedicine allows real-time consultation with the event location and emergency department and coronary care unit. Early trials of telemedicine systems show that clinical information can be viewed in real-time, with transfer of a 12-lead ECG at 60-second intervals. This will give general practitioners unprecedented access to specialist advice.[15] Although widely used in Europe, the prehospital ECG has seen only limited use in Brazil.

Telemedicine Programs in Brazil

Research studies from around the world have established the efficacy of telemedicine versus standard measures for reducing mortality in the management of AMI.[16] The relative risk for in-hospital mortality from AMI was 0.65 (95% confidence interval, 0.42–0.99) for the telemedicine group compared with the usual care group, thus showing the benefit of telemedicine for AMI patients. Obtaining ECGs during the prehospital period may improve the health outcomes in patients with coronary artery disease.

The basic telemedicine program in Brazil is part of the National Program for Emergency and Urgency established in 2003. Every chest pain patient has an ECG registered and transmitted to a telemedicine center, where cardiologists are available 24 hours/7 days. If the patient is triaged, he is transferred to a PPCI. When logistics are not favorable, tenecteplase is given in the ambulance and the patient is transferred to a hospital.

Concerns still exist, however, regarding the best means for providing real-time field interpretation of the prehospital ECG and the potential for inappropriate field time delay, triage, and treatment of patients. Moreover, questions remain about the overall clinical and cost benefit of expanding this resource universally.[17]

CURRENT PROGRAMS—SAMU

In 2003, the Ministry of Health of Brazil launched the National Program for Emergency and Urgency to structure and organize the network of emergency departments in the country. Because the publication of the ordinance and establishing this policy, the goal has been to coordinate emergency services that lead up to attention at the ED.[18] SAMU performs accident and emergency services at any location: houses, work areas, and public roads. The service works 24 hours a day with teams of doctors, nurses, nursing assistants, and first aid specialists, who attend traumatic events, clinics, pediatrics, surgeries, obstetrics and gynecology, and mental health needs of the population. Help comes via a free call to the telephone number 192. The call is answered by technicians who identify the emergency and transfer the call to a doctor. The doctor diagnoses the situation and starts attendance at the same time, advising the patient or the person who made the call regarding first aid. Depending on the patient's situation, the doctor may advise the person to go to a health station, send an ambulance to the area with the help of a nurse or first-aid specialist, or send a mobile intensive care unit (UTIM), with a doctor or nurse. Simultaneously, the doctor offers advice regarding the closest public hospital so that quick treatment can continue.

The different units and interventions available at SAMU are:

- Basic Life Support Units: Each Mobile Basic Support Unit has a tele-electrocardiograph and a manual resuscitator.
- UTIM: Each UTIM has at least the following equipment: a volume respirator, a multiparameter monitor, a tele-electrocardiograph, a pulse oximeter, and digital syringe infusion pump, as well as all the material for immobilization and intensive care medicine.
- Helicopter Advanced Life Support: The helicopter advanced life support, made possible through an agreement between the Federal Highway Police and SAMU, is equipped with at least: a surgical aspirator, a volume respirator, a multiparameter monitor, a tele-electrocardiographer, a digital oximeter, and syringe infusion pump, as well as all the material for immobilization and intensive care medicine.

UTIMs are equipped with digital and nondigital 12-lead tele-electrocardiographs with the capacity of transmitting the ECG tracings through landlines, mobile phones, and computers, and forwarding the results to an on-duty cardiologist. The entire process of transmitting data from the ECG device to a mobile phone or device and obtain the diagnosis from the cardiologist takes an average of 5 minutes. UTIMs are physician manned. The Basic Life Support Units are paramedic manned and not equipped with the tele-ECG system.

CONCLUSION

During the past 50 years, health systems have evolved to reduce in-hospital AMI mortality, reducing it from 30% in the 1960s to 4% in the 2009.[12] Unfortunately, prehospital mortality has not changed during the same period and nowadays it accounts for almost 75% of total the AMI mortality rate throughout the world. Data from DATASUS shows that prehospital mortality is 50% in Brazil.[14]

The Brazilian Society of Cardiology has created a national program to promote a better and universal treatment for AMI by means of an educational effort to improve awareness of key information for prehospital approach that must start at the place where the patient experiences the first symptom.[19] The Ministry of Health published its guidelines for ACS,[20] strengthening the importance of prehospital ECG and thrombolysis, as well as rapid transfer to PCI-capable centers, when appropriate. There are 2502 mobile prehospital units, among them 1324 SAMU ambulances, registered at the Ministry of Health database.[18]

The government is aware of the disability-adjusted life-year impact on global health performance and how a well-developed prehospital approach can change this scenario in poor areas of the country. A recent analysis of prehospital care for stroke and AMI in the elderly population of Minas Gerais, Brazil, suggests that the National Urgent Care Policy has not yet been able to achieve its goals.[21] As an example, the AMI mortality rate for a Rio de Janeiro nears 26.7 deaths per 100 during prehospital care; however, mortality reaches 66% in the south area of the city.[22]

Brazil healthcare has evolved over the past 15 years supported by the economic growth, narrowing of the inequalities, health budget growth, and technological improvement. The prehospital environment has experienced dramatic change, with the implementation of SAMU and telemedicine for prehospital ECG transmission and thrombolysis. Efforts continue to improve the availability of this service throughout the country. However, effective coverage of 5564 cities that are dispersed across more than 8 billion km^2 is not an easy task for any health system.

REFERENCES

1. Fletcher GF, Balady GJ, Vogel RA, et al. 33rd Bethesda Conference: Preventive Cardiology: How can we do better? *J Am Coll Cardiol.* 2002;40(4):579–651.
2. Síntese de Indicadores Sociais 2006. Estudos e Pesquisas. Informação demográfica e Socioeconômica número 19. Ministério do Planejamento, Orçamento e Gestão, Instituto Brasileiro de Geografia e Estatística – IBGE, Diretoria de Pesquisas Coordenação de População e Indicadores Sociais. Available at: http://www.ibge.gov.br/home/estatistica/populacao/condicaodevida/indicadoresminimos/sinteseindicsociais2006/indicsociais2006.pdf. Accessed June 17, 2007.
3. Cadastro Nacional de Estabelecimentos de Saúde. CNES Net. Secretaria de Atenção à Saúde. DATASUS. Tipos de estabelecimentos. Available at: http://cnes.datasus.gov.br/Mod_Ind_Unidade.asp?VEstado=00 Accessed on March 28, 2013.
4. Mattos LA. Infarto Agudo do Miocárdio: Atendimento Pré-hospitalar e Angioplastia Facilitada. Available at: http://www.sohcierj.org.br/arquivos/Aulas/X_Simposio_Sohcierj/aulas_pdf/Luiz_Matos.pdf. Accessed on March 26, 2013.
5. Número de profissionais de saúde por habitante. Indicadores de Recurso. Rede interagencial de Informações para a Saúde. Available

at: http://tabnet.datasus.gov.br/cgi/tabcgi.exe?idb2006/e01.def. Accessed on June 17, 2007.

6. Orçamento Annual de 2013. Projeto de Lei Orçamentária Annual – PLOA 2013. Ministério do Planejamento, Orçamento e Gestão. Available at: http://www.planejamento.gov.br/secretaria.asp?cat=50&sub=654&sec=8. Accessed on March 28, 2013.
7. Mobile Emergency Service. SAMU. Available at: http://www.brasil.gov.br/sobre/health/service/samu. Accessed on March 27, 2013.
8. Marcos K, Marcelo N, Adriana P, Elias K. Unidade de Dor Torácica: importância no tratamento da síndrome isquêmica aguda com supradesnivelamento do segmento ST. *Rev Soc Cardiol Estado de São Paulo.* 2004;6:887–892.
9. Polanczyk CA, Kuntz K, Sacks DB, et al. Cost-effectiveness of triage strategies using CK-MB and troponin I in emergency department patients with acute chest pain. *Ann Intern Med.* 1999;131:909–918.
10. Damasceno CA, Mussi FC. Prehospital delay factors in myocardial infarction: a literature review. *Cienc Cuid Saude.* 2010;9(4):815–821.
11. Goldberg RJ, Steg PG, Sadiq I, et al. Extent of, and factors associated with, delay to hospital presentation in patients with acute coronary disease (The GRACE Registry). *Am J Cardiol.* 2002;89(7):791–796.
12. McGovern PG, Pankow JS, Shahar E, et al. The Minnesota Heart Survey Investigators. Recent trends in acute coronary heart disease. *N Engl J Med.* 1996;334:884–890.
13. Mansur AP, Souza MFM, Favarato D, et al. Stroke and ischemic heart disease mortality trends in Brazil from 1979 to 1996. *Neuroepidemiology.* 2003;22:179–183.
14. Linha de cuidado do infarto agudo do miocárdio na rede de atenção às urgências. Available at: http://www.saude.pr.gov.br/arquivos/File/HOSPSUS/protocolo_sindrome_coronariaMS2011.pdf. Accessed on September 2, 2014.
15. Karagounis L, Ipsen SK, Jessop MR, et al. Impact of field-transmitted electrocardiography on time to in-hospital thrombolytic therapy in acute myocardial infarction. *Am J Cardiol.* 1990;66:786–791.
16. De Waure C, Cadeddu C, Gualano MR, Ricciardi W. Telemedicine for the reduction of myocardial infarction mortality: A systematic review and a meta-analysis of published studies. *Telemed J E Health.* 2012;18(5):323–328.
17. Canto JG, Rogers WJ, Bowlby LJ, et al. The prehospital electrocardiogram in acute myocardial infarction: Is its full potential being realized? National Registry of Myocardial Infarction 2 Investigators. *J Am Coll Cardiol.* 1997;29:498–505.
18. Mobile Emergency Service. SAMU. Available at: http://www.brasil.gov.br/sobre/health/service/samu. Accessed on March 27, 2013.
19. Coracao Alerta. Available at: www.coracaoalerta.com.br/campanha. Accessed on March 28, 2013.

20. Consulta Pública número 6 de 20 de Setembro de 2011. Available at: http://www.saude.gov.br/sas.
21. Luz Cde, Junger WL, Cavalini LT. Analysis of prehospital care for stroke and acute myocardial infarction in the elderly population of Minas Gerais, Brazil. *Rev Assoc Med Bras*. 2010;56(4):452–456.
22. Tempo-resposta das ambulâncias para casos graves e as taxas de mortalidade nos bairros. Available at: http://extra.globo.com/noticias/rio/confira-tempo-resposta-das-ambulancias-para-graves-as-taxas-de-mortalidade-nos-bairros-5121795.html#ixzz2Ogo5SwAs. Accessed on March 27, 2013.

CHAPTER 12

Chile: Prehospital Management of STEMI

Edgardo Escobar, MD

DEMOGRAPHICS AND EPIDEMIOLOGY

Chile has 16,634,603 inhabitants (2012), with 30% of them living in Santiago, the capital. The ratio of physicians to inhabitants is reasonable, 1:559; however, there is an uneven distribution, with a high percentage of physicians practicing in Santiago. Additionally, there are a limited number of cardiovascular specialists and extensive rural areas.

Cardiovascular diseases (CVDs) are the main causes of death with 29% of total mortality, 31% of which are due to coronary heart disease and 32% to cerebrovascular disease. Acute myocardial infarction (AMI) is the first cause of death (36/100,000 in 2006).

According to a survey of the Ministry of Health performed in 2009/2010 among 5434 adults aged 15 years or older, 27% of the population is hypertensive, 9.4% have diabetes, 53% are smokers, 25% are obese, 38% have dyslipidemia, and 88% are sedentary. These figures are even worse than the same survey performed in 2003.[1]

CVDs are one of the three most common causes of disability (average age of 49 years for women and 53 for men).[2] Facing this scenario. the Ministry of Health has implemented a Cardiovascular Health Program, details of which are beyond

Prehospital Management of Acute STEMI: Practical Approaches and International Strategies for Early Intervention © 2015 Joseph S. Alpert, Lynne T. Braun, Barbara J. Fletcher, Gerald Fletcher, Editors-in-Chief, Cardiotext Publishing, ISBN: 978-1-935395-66-9

the scope of this analysis. Suffice it to say that at the primary care level, the goals are well defined and periodically supervised by health authorities. On the other hand, there have been important political decisions, namely a very strict antismoking law, a nutritional education program, and a law called Acceso Universal con Garantías Explícitas (AUGE; Universal Access with Explicit Guarantees).[3] According to this law, the health-care system has the obligation to take care of 80 diseases in a predetermined period of time. For example, if hypertension or diabetes is diagnosed, the patient has to be under treatment no later than 7 days. As a result of the AUGE, several important steps to standardize systems of ST-elevation myocardial infarction (STEMI) care have been implemented, which are described in more detail below.

ACCESS TO MEDICAL ASSISTANCE

Patients have two main routes for obtaining medical assistance: mobile emergency care (SAMU) activated by calling the 131 phone number, or going directly to an emergency primary service (SAPU). The SAMU is an ambulance with medical and paramedical personnel, able to deliver emergency care, including tracheal intubation. They transport the patient either to SAPUs, which are facilities spread all over the country, with the capability to transmit the ECG to the central call center and to perform thrombolysis, or directly to a reference hospital as defined by the Ministry of Health.

A patient with chest pain suggestive of an acute coronary event must have an ECG ideally within 10 minutes.

NATIONAL ECG CALL CENTER

Since May 1, 2004, the Ministry of Health implemented national coverage of ECG telemedicine for the purpose of diagnostic interpretation and the possibility of performing thrombolysis even in rural areas. The 12-lead ECG is acquired in SAPUs or the emergency room of a hospital and transmitted by phone, even by cell phone, or internet to a central call center. There is only one ECG call center for the entire country, based in the capital.

The call center is staffed with paramedics and specialists on a 24/7 basis, and technical service is provided by a private company, International Telemedical System SA (ITMS). It was recognized by the Ministry of Health as being able to provide the diagnostic support for STEMI and increasing options for SAPU physicians to perform thrombolysis 24 hours a day, 365 days a year.

ITMS receives ECGs from all over the country on a 24/7 basis. The ECGS are received by trained paramedics in a computer. If they are technically correct, after recording all the clinical and demographic data, they are transmitted to the doctor's computer. Those ECGs with ST-segment elevation, as recognized by the paramedics in their computers, have absolute priority and should be further interpreted by a cardiologist within 10 minutes.[4] Figure 12.1 shows this telemedicine system of ECG interpretation coordinated with the central role of con sultation by the cardiologist on duty.

CARDIOLOGY CONSULTANT CONTACT WITH PRIMARY PHYSICIANS

All SAPU are equipped with transmission devices through which they transmit all chest pain consultations. The report of STEMI is sent back to the place of origin and to the hospital of reference according to the network defined by the Ministry of Health, where primary percutaneous coronary intervention (PPCI) or thrombolysis is performed if PPCI is not available on-site. In addition, by ITMS protocol the cardiologist on duty

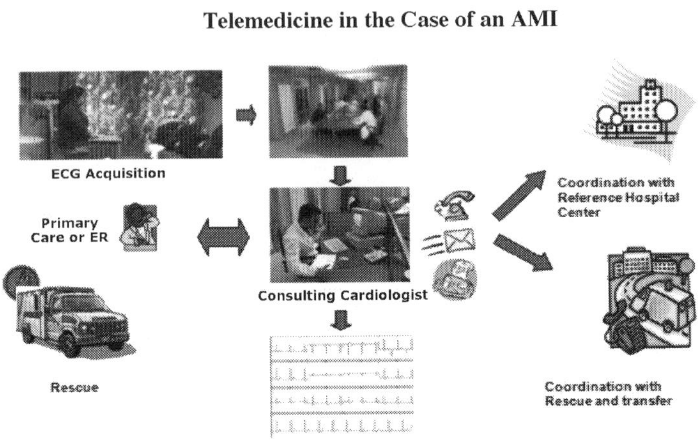

Figure 12.1

Telemedicine and cardiology consultation in the case of AMI. ECG acquired on site is sent by phone or internet to a central station, where it is accepted by trained paramedic personnel, and a report made by cardiologists. The report is sent back to the place of origin and to the hospital of reference.

has to make telephone contact with the doctor in charge to confirm the diagnosis and give advice if necessary.

NATIONAL PROTOCOL FOR THROMBOLYSIS

The Ministry of Health, with the support of the Chilean Society of Cardiology, outlined a protocol which must be followed all over the country (Figure 12.2).[5]

According to this protocol, thrombolysis with streptokinase should be started ideally within 3 hours after diagnosis, provided that there is no the possibility of sending the patient for PPCI within 90 minutes of first medical contact (FMC). This strategy gives priority to "time to accurate diagnosis," which is different than other approaches, for 2 reasons: the AUGE law and the interpretation of the ECG made by cardiologists. It has

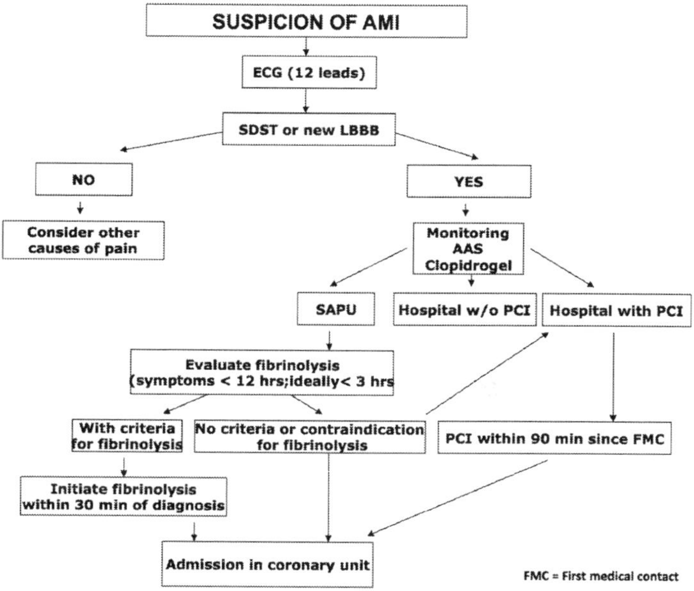

Figure 12.2

Algorithm for the Ministry of Health national protocol for diagnosis and treatment of STEMI. Spanish abbreviations: SDST, ST elevation; AAS, aspirin.

been shown that teletransmission of an ECG before hospital admission can greatly accelerate in-hospital management and increase the probability of timely reperfusion therapy.[6,7]

THE AUGE LAW AND PATIENT OUTCOMES FOR AMI

The impact of the AUGE law in improving outcomes for patients with AMI was evaluated. A total of 3547 patients with AMI were analyzed in 9 hospitals, 2623 pre-AUGE and 924 after the law was instituted.[8] Time between initiation of symptoms and admission was 4 hours in both periods, with only 25% of patients admitted before 3 hours. Time between admission and thrombolysis was 31 minutes. Global mortality at 30 days decreased from 12% to 8.6% (odds ratio = 0.64, adjusted by age, gender, risk factors, previous MI, and Killip score at admission). There was a greater mortality reduction in higher-risk patients (women and patients older than 75 years). In patients treated with thrombolysis, mortality decreased from 10.6% to 6.8% ($P < 0.0005$), even in places with low complexity of care.

Although the time delay between initiation of symptoms and FMC has not improved, the decrease in mortality can be explained by the increased rates of thrombolysis from 50% to 61% and PPCI from 2.3% to 7.3%. There have also been significant increases in the prescription of statins, β-blockers, angiotensin converting enzyme inhibitors (ACEIs), and aspirin.[8]

CONCLUSION

In summary, there have been important advances in Chile in the care of patients with AMI, improving early diagnosis and treatment through the telemedicine system as an important support. Telemedicine is an important tool for the interpretation of the prehospital ECG, particularly if there is a central station of report, as in the case of Chile, to initiate treatment on-site or to activate the whole system.[9] The combination of public policies (AUGE law) and private efforts has proved to be very successful. The Strategic Reperfusion Early After Myocardial Infarction (STREAM) trial gives support to the strategy of treatment in Chile, demonstrating that early thrombolysis with tenecteplase can benefit STEMI patients who cannot undergo PPCI within the first hour of medical contact.[10]

REFERENCES

1. Encuesta Nacional de Salud, ENS, Chile, 2009/2010. Ministerio de Salud, Gobierno de Chile. Minsal.cl.

2. Ministerio de Salud de Chile. Available at: http://epi.minsal.cl/epi/html/ivest/cargaenf2008/minuta21-07-2008.pdf.
3. AUGE. Available at: http://web.minsal.cl/AUGE_INTRODUCCION.
4. Escobar E, Véjar M, del Pino R. Lesiones subepicárdicas en Chile (Infarto agudo del miocardio con supradesnivel del segmento ST). Experiencia con telemedicina. *Rev Chil Cardiol.* 2009;28:73–80.
5. Guías Clínicas. Available at: http://www.minsal.cl.
6. Thygesen K, Alpert JS, Jaffe AS, et al. Third universal definition of myocardial infarction. *Eur Heart J.* 2012;33:2551–2567.
7. Quinn T, Johnsen S, Gale CP, et al. Effects of prehospital 12-lead ECG on process of care and morality in acute coronary syndrome; a linked cohort study from the myocardial ischaemia National Audit Project. *Heart.* 2014;100(12):944–950.
8. Nassal NC, Campos TP, Corbalán R, et al. Grupo GEMI, Departamento de estudios multicéntricos, Sociedad Chilena de Cardiología y Cirugía Cardiovascular. Impacto del plan AUGE en el tratamiento de pacientes con Infarto Agudo al Miocardio con supradesnivel del segmento ST en hospitales chilenos. *Rev Med Chile.* 2008;136:1231–1239.
9. Sorensen JTH, Clemmensen P, Sjersten M. Telecardiologia: Pasado, presente y future. *Rev Esp Cardiol.* 2013;66:212–218.
10. Armstrong PW, Gershlick AH, Goldstein P, et al. STREAM investigative team. Fibrinolysis or primary PCI in ST segment elevation myocardial infarction. *N Engl J Med.* 2013;368:1379–1387.

CHAPTER 13

France: Prehospital Management of STEMI

Nicolas Danchin, MD, PhD, Etienne Puymirat, MD, Eric Durand, MD, PhD, and Patrick Goldstein, MD

INTRODUCTION

Prehospital management of acute myocardial infarction (AMI) in France is organized under the supervision of an extremely well-developed network of mobile intensive care units (MICUs) under the banner of the nationwide Service d'Aide Médicale Urgente (SAMU).[1] The first local SAMU was created 47 years ago in 1968 in Toulouse, and it took more than 10 years for the SAMU to create an emergency call number available for the general population. Following this initial experience, the current nationwide organization of the SAMU was organized in 1986, with one local SAMU for each county ("département"), and a common national call number, 15. Each local SAMU is headed by an emergency physician, and is organized with a medical response center, which receives emergency calls from the public 24/7 and decides upon the optimal way to manage each specific situation. In addition, each SAMU has several local MICUs based at different regional hospitals, to offer the shortest possible delays to access the patients in need of emergency care. There are about 1000 MICUs in France, in a network of 106 local SAMUs.

Prehospital Management of Acute STEMI: Practical Approaches and International Strategies for Early Intervention © 2015 Joseph S. Alpert, Lynne T. Braun, Barbara J. Fletcher, Gerald Fletcher, Editors-in-Chief, Cardiotext Publishing, ISBN: 978-1-935395-66-9

GENERAL SCHEME OF PREHOSPITAL MANAGEMENT OF SUSPECTED AMI

In the case of acute chest pain or symptoms suggestive of possible acute coronary syndrome (ACS), the physician answering the call will dispatch a medically staffed ambulance (including a physician) to the patient's location; in some cases, when conditions are such that ground transportation would be impossible or unacceptably long, a medically staffed helicopter may be sent to the site. By law, MICUs are required to be staffed by a physician trained in emergency medicine, a nurse, and a driver trained in cardiopulmonary resuscitation. Physicians participate in regular training sessions to improve their knowledge of ECG interpretation. This interprofessional team is capable of a wide range of therapeutic options for prehospital management for acute coronary care and AMI.

Once on site, the MICU team will perform the first diagnostic ECG and based upon the findings, then the optimal therapeutic management will be decided. In the case of ST-elevation myocardial infarction (STEMI), the medical response center will determine the location of the nearest hospital offering 24/7 percutaneous coronary intervention (PCI) capability and contact it to determine catheterization laboratory availability. Depending on the patient's characteristics and condition, distances, and expected traffic, the emergency physician will decide whether to use immediate prehospital fibrinolytic treatment or to bring the patient to a catheterization laboratory to perform primary percutaneous coronary intervention (PPCI).

EVALUATION AND PROGRESS OF PREHOSPITAL AMI MANAGEMENT IN FRANCE

Since 1995, a nationwide program for the purpose of monitoring the way patients with AMI are managed has been organized

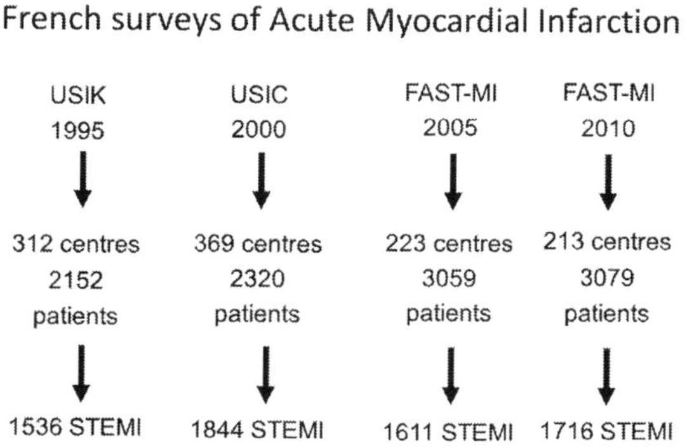

Figure 13.1

French surveys for monitoring AMI management from 1995 to 2010.

in France.[2-5] All patients with STEMI or non-ST-elevation myocardial infarction (NSTEMI) are included, if the onset of symptoms is ≤48 hours from hospitalization (Figure 13.1). This program is based upon one-month surveys, which are set up every 5 years in voluntary hospitals taking care of AMI patients; participation rates have varied from 60% to 80% of all French institutions, be it academic hospitals, general public hospitals, private clinics, and army hospitals. Data on prehospital use of fibrinolytic therapy have been recorded since the 2000 survey, and detailed information on prehospital management has been recorded in the 2005 and 2010 surveys.

Patient Use of the SAMU for Initial Medical Contact

In the Unité de Soins Intensifs Coronaires (USIC) 2000 survey, first medical contact was through SAMU in 27% of the cases for patients with STEMI or a new Q wave seen within 12 hours of symptom onset. However, the proportion of patients transported by the SAMU was 61%, because in many instances the first medical party involved subsequently called the SAMU.

In the Acute ST-elevation and Non-ST-elevation Myocardial Infarction (FAST-MI) 2005 French registry, the proportion of patients initially calling the SAMU had increased to 45%, and a total of 63% were transported by the SAMU; while 30% of the patients initially called their general practitioner, and 15% of patients presented directly to the emergency room. In the FAST-MI 2010 registry, the proportion of patients initially calling the SAMU had increased to 53% and a total of 84% were transported by the SAMU (Figure 13.2). Beyond 12 hours following symptom onset, the proportion of patients transported by the SAMU also notably increased from 2000 (10%) to 2005 (39%) and to 2010 (65%), in relation with a more frequent utilization of MICUs as a secondary intervening party (22% in 2000 and 2005, and 51% in 2010). In addition to the increased use of the SAMU as the first intervening party, patient delay

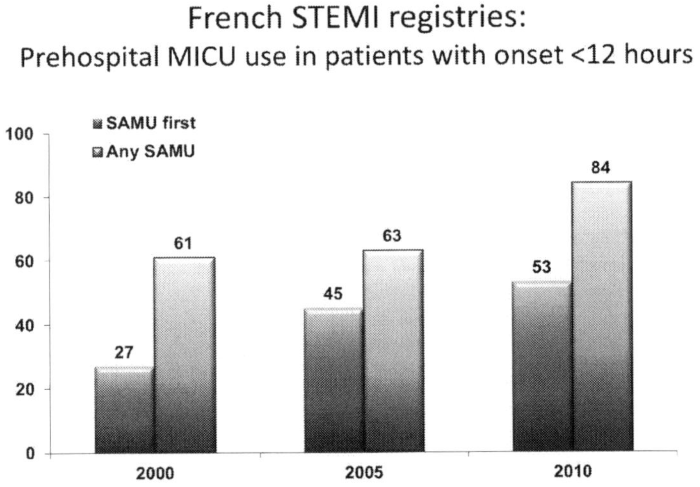

Figure 13.2

Percentage of STEMI patients making use of the SAMU as the first intervening party or at any time before hospital admission. MICU is the French designation for the transportation section of the SAMU. Data from the USIC 2000 and FAST-MI 2005 and 2010 registries.

from symptom onset to first call also decreased. In the whole STEMI population, median time from symptom onset to first call decreased from 120 minutes in 2000 to 90 minutes in 2005 and 74 minutes in 2010; for the patients who directly called the SAMU, median time from symptom onset to call also decreased from 75 minutes in 1995 to 60 minutes in 2005 and 45 minutes in 2010.

Both in 2005 and 2010, patients initially calling the SAMU were less frequently admitted to the emergency room, once reaching the hospital (37% in 2005, versus 63% for those not calling the SAMU first, and 30% in 2010, versus 65% when the SAMU was not called first). Instead, most patients were brought directly to the ICCU and others directly to the cath lab.

Typology of STEMI Patients by Using the SAMU for Initial Call and Regional Variations in Usage

The typology of STEMI patients in relation to initial pathway has been studied in the FAST-MI 2010 registry. An initial call to the SAMU was more frequent in current smokers (53% vs. 46%), in patients with a history of coronary artery disease (52.5% vs. 45%), as well as for patients calling within 2 hours of symptom onset (59.5% vs. 31.5%), or those with an initial cardiac arrest or syncope (81.5% vs. 48%) or Killip class III or more at the time of admission (66% vs. 48%). Other demographics such as age and gender were similar in those having called the SAMU first and those using other pathways. Likewise, the presence of diabetes mellitus, hypertension, hypercholesterolemia, or family history did not significantly differ. Independent correlates of initial call to the SAMU are listed in Table 13.1.

In addition to these differences in patient profile, important regional variations in the use of SAMU as the first intervening party were noted: the SAMU was the most often used

Table 13.1
Independent correlates of initial call to the SAMU by using multivariate logistic regression in the FAST-MI 2010 registry

	OR (95% CI)	*P* value
Chest pain ≤120 min	3.30 (2.64–4.12)	<0.001
Onset during weekend	1.47 (1.16–1.86)	0.002
Onset during night	1.54 (1.21–1.95)	<0.001
Cardiac arrest/syncope	1.94 (1.30–2.91)	0.001
Intensity of chest pain ≥7/10	1.51 (1.07–2.13)	0.02
Current smoking	1.34 (1.08–1.66)	0.008
No history of CAD	0.71 (0.54–0.94)	0.02

CAD, coronary artery disease; OR, odds ratio.

in Paris and suburbs (59%), and the least in the rural center region (37%).

Use of Prehospital Fibrinolysis and Reperfusion Therapy

In patients who called the SAMU first, major changes in the use and type of reperfusion therapy have been observed in the past years (Figure 13.3).[6,7] In patients with time from symptom onset to first call ≤12 hours, PPCI was stable from 2000 to 2005, but increased considerably from 2005 (39%) to 2010 (69.3%). This change was most probably related to the reduction in the number of institutions taking care of STEMI patients, following recommendations of the French health authorities, with more patients being directly admitted to institutions with PCI capability. Prehospital fibrinolytic treatment was used in 21% of the patients in 2000, it increased to 33% in 2005, and subsequently markedly decreased to 14% in 2010. In-hospital use of fibrinolysis consistently decreased from 18% to 7% and 4% over the same time period. Important changes

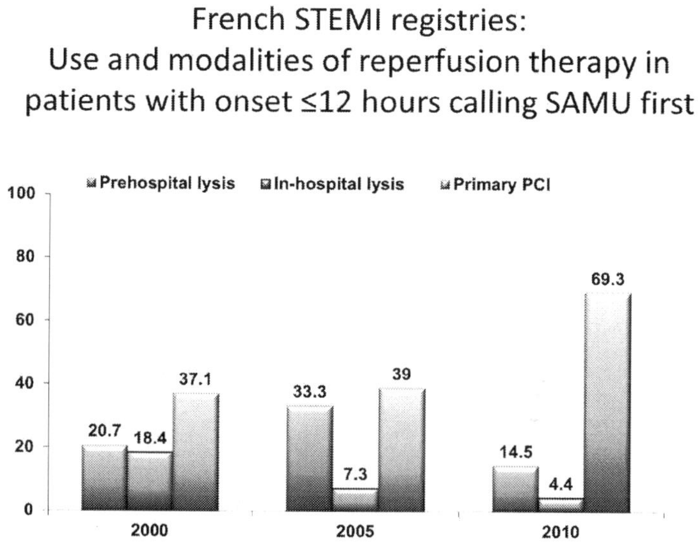

Figure 13.3

Modalities of reperfusion therapy in STEMI patients initially calling the SAMU: Evolution from 2000 to 2010.

were also observed in the type of fibrinolytic treatment used: in 2000, 67% of the patients received alteplase, 22% reteplase, 5% streptokinase, and 5% tenecteplase, but in 2005 and 2010, only fibrin-specific agents were used. In 2005, tenecteplase was used in 78% (likely because of its easier use), alteplase in 13.5% and reteplase in 6%, and in 2010, tenecteplase was used in 91.5% of the patients.

Other Procedures and Medications

Among patients for whom the SAMU was called first, 5% had cardiopulmonary resuscitation, and 1% needed tracheal intubation before hospital admission. The STEMI diagnosis was correctly recognized in the field in 97% of the patients, while 3% were initially considered to have non-ST elevation-acute coronary syndrome (NSTE-ACS); in contrast, among patients who did not use the SAMU, 11% were initially considered to have NSTE-ACS. In patients who were transported by the SAMU, the initially intended reperfusion strategy was fibrinolysis in 19%, PPCI in 69%, and no urgent reperfusion therapy in 12%. Subsequent to this initially chosen proposed strategy, fibrinolysis was actually used in 99% of the intended patients and PPCI in 87%. On the other hand, 67% of those in whom no reperfusion therapy was initially proposed actually underwent emergent coronary angiography, and of these, 52% actually underwent PPCI.

Of the patients initially transported by the SAMU in 2010, 72% received aspirin in the ambulance, 56% clopidogrel (52% of these had a 300 mg loading dose and 42% a 600 mg or more loading dose), 11.5% received prasugrel (97% with a 60 mg loading dose), and 5% had intravenous glycoprotein IIb–IIIa receptor blockers. The most commonly used anticoagulant was unfractionated heparin (36%), while low molecular weight heparin was used in 30%. Other medications included nitrates (25%), loop diuretics (2%), intravenous inotropes (2%), anxiolytics (3.5%), β-blockers (1%), opioids (30.5%), and other analgesics or sedatives (25%). The use of adjunct therapies during transportation by the SAMU increased from 2005 to 2010 (Table 13.2).

EARLY OUTCOMES ACCORDING TO PREHOSPITAL USE OF MEDICATIONS AND PROCEDURES

Prehospital Fibrinolysis

The outcomes in patients treated with prehospital fibrinolysis have been studied in the USIC 2000 registry.[8,9] Patients treated with fibrinolytics prehospital were younger (59 years vs. 61 years) and more often men than women. In-hospital mortality was 3.3% in those receiving prehospital fibrinolysis,

Table 13.2
Prehospital adjunct therapies for STEMI in SAMU-transported patients

Use of Medications in Ambulance	2005 (%)	2010 (%)
Aspirin	62	72
Clopidogrel	16	56
Prasugrel	–	11.5
GP IIb-IIIa blocker	4	5
UFH	42	36
LMWH	18	30
Morphine	28	30.5
IV nitrates	33	25
β-blockers	3	1

GP, glycoprotein; LMWH, low molecular weight heparin; UFH, unfractionated heparin.

compared with 6.7% for PPCI and 8.0% for in-hospital fibrinolysis. Likewise, one-year mortality tended to be lower (hazard ratio adjusted on baseline parameters: 0.49, 95% confidence interval: 0.24–1.00, $P = 0.05$).

Similar trends were found in the FAST-MI 2005 registry.[10] At that time, intravenous fibrinolysis was no longer used as a stand-alone therapy, but rather as the initial part of a pharmacoinvasive strategy: early fibrinolysis, followed by later coronary angiography and routine PCI when possible (84% of the patients underwent PCI after fibrinolysis). Using propensity-score matching, one-year survival was 94% for patients initially receiving fibrinolysis, compared with 93% for PPCI.

Prehospital Antithrombotic Medications

The impact of prehospital antithrombotic medications outside the use of fibrinolytic treatment was also analyzed in the FAST-MI 2010 survey. Prehospital medications were used more frequently in patients who had called within one hour of symptom onset, compared with those having called later; the respective figures were 69.5% versus 54% for aspirin, 52% versus 42% for clopidogrel, 13% versus 8% for prasugrel, 63% versus 48% for administration of dual antiplatelet therapy, and 63% versus 49% for the use of any type of anticoagulant.

Thirty-day mortality was lower when antithrombotic medications were administered in the ambulance for this same group of patients who called within 60 minutes of symptom onset (1.5% vs. 6.1%, respectively, for patients with or without dual antiplatelet therapy; 1.4% vs. 6.4%, respectively, for those with or without heparin therapy, $P < 0.001$). In contrast, only a trend persisted in favor of the early administration of antithrombotic treatment when time from symptom onset to call was greater than one hour.

Finally, the FAST-MI 2010 data confirmed the importance of avoiding time delays for patients undergoing PPCI. Median time from ECG to PPCI in patients having called the SAMU was 100 minutes, and 25% of the population had a time delay greater than 144 minutes, thus by far exceeding current recommendations. In-hospital mortality was notably and significantly lower in patients in whom the recommended timelines for performing PPCI were followed (1.5% vs. 3.8%). Overall, getting reperfusion therapy (either by PPCI or fibrinolysis) beyond recommended thresholds was an independent predictor of higher in-hospital mortality (odds ratio: 3.12, 95% confidence interval: 1.10–8.85).

CONCLUSION

Nationally organized surveys in France have been systematically collecting data on prehospital AMI management and outcomes since 1995. Several important trends have emerged that point to both successes and areas for improvement.

Public education and utilization: In spite of the availability of a well-developed and recognized MICU network for medical transportation, the French SAMU is used as the first contact with medical care by little more than 50% STEMI patients; it is, however, used by 5 out of 6 patients when secondary transportation is taken into account.

An encouraging increase in the use of the national emergency call number was found from 2000 to 2010, most likely related to repeated public information campaigns involving the press, radio, and television.

Guideline implementation: Although increasing, the use of recommended antithrombotic medications (anticoagulants, aspirin, and thienopyridines) in the prehospital setting is still far from 100%, reflecting the difficulties encountered in implementing guidelines in the real world.

Ongoing concerns with the time delay to PPCI: Finally, one may wonder whether the recent decrease in the use of prehospital fibrinolysis is justified, as about one third of patients undergoing PPCI still have their intervention performed beyond currently recommended timelines, with a related increase in early mortality. In fact, our "real-world" data lead us to recommend remembering that, when used in a timely fashion in patients without contraindications and as part of a pharmacoinvasive strategy, intravenous fibrinolysis should be the preferred reperfusion therapy when guidelines-recommended timing of PPCI is unlikely to be achieved.

REFERENCES

1. Cara M. [Emergency medical assistance and organization of emergency medical care units in France (SAMU)]. *Ann Pharmaceut Franc.* 2002;60(4):219–225.
2. Cambou JP, Simon T, Mulak G, Bataille V, Danchin N. The French registry of Acute ST elevation or non-ST-elevation Myocardial Infarction (FAST-MI): Study design and baseline characteristics. *Arch Mal Coeur Vaiss.* 2007;100(6–7):524–534.

3. Danchin N, Vaur L, Genes N, et al. Management of acute myocardial infarction in intensive care units in 1995: A nationwide French survey of practice and early hospital results. *J Am Coll Cardiol.* 1997;30(7):1598–1605.
4. Hanania G, Cambou JP, Gueret P, et al. Management and in-hospital outcome of patients with acute myocardial infarction admitted to intensive care units at the turn of the century: Results from the French nationwide USIC 2000 registry. *Heart.* 2004;90(12):1404–1410.
5. Hanssen M, Cottin Y, Khalife K, et al. French Registry on Acute ST-elevation and non ST-elevation Myocardial Infarction 2010. FAST-MI 2010. *Heart.* 2012;98(9):699–705.
6. Danchin N. Systems of care for ST-segment elevation myocardial infarction: Impact of different models on clinical outcomes. *JACC Cardiovasc Interv.* 2009;2(10):901–908.
7. Puymirat E, Simon T, Steg PG, et al. Association of changes in clinical characteristics and management with improvement in survival among patients with ST-elevation myocardial infarction. *JAMA.* 2012;308(10):998–1006.
8. Danchin N, Blanchard D, Steg PG, et al. Impact of prehospital thrombolysis for acute myocardial infarction on 1-year outcome: Results from the French Nationwide USIC 2000 Registry. *Circulation.* 2004;110(14):1909–1915.
9. Danchin N, Durand E, Blanchard D. Pre-hospital thrombolysis in perspective. *Eur Heart J.* 2008;29(23):2835–2842.
10. Danchin N, Coste P, Ferrieres J, et al. Comparison of thrombolysis followed by broad use of percutaneous coronary intervention with primary percutaneous coronary intervention for ST-segment-elevation acute myocardial infarction: Data from the french registry on acute ST-elevation myocardial infarction (FAST-MI). *Circulation.* 2008;118(3):268–276.

Index

Page numbers followed by *f*, *t*, refer to figures, tables

A

D

E

R

S

T

U

W